the
fine art of
DRESSING

the fine art of DRESSING

Make Yourself a Masterpiece by
Dressing for Your Body Type

Margaux Tartarotti

Illustrations by the author

A PERIGEE BOOK

A Perigee Book
Published by The Berkley Publishing Group
A division of Penguin Putnam Inc.
375 Hudson Street
New York, New York 10014

First edition: January 2000

Published simultaneously in Canada.

The Penguin Putnam Inc. World Wide Web site address is http://www.penguinputnam.com

Library of Congress Cataloging-in-Publication Data

Tartarotti, Margaux.
The fine art of dressing: make yourself a masterpiece by dressing for your body type /
by Margaux Tartarotti.
p. cm.
Includes index.
ISBN 0-399-52568-8
1. Clothing and dress. 2. Fashion. I. Title.

TT507 .T37 1999
646'.34—dc21
99-046120
CIP

Printed in the United States of America

10 9 8 7 6 5 4 3 2 1

To my family

CONTENTS

acknowledgments

I wish to express my thanks to all those who contributed to the development of this book, especially Evelyn Lessem and Yves Rouffignac, and also Heidi Leverty, Anne Game, and Stefan Chiarantano.

Grateful appreciation goes to:
John Duff, Dolores McMullan, Erin Stryker, and Charles Björklund, at Perigee, a division of Penguin Putnam Inc.

Finally, I thank my family and friends for their support and enthusiasm.

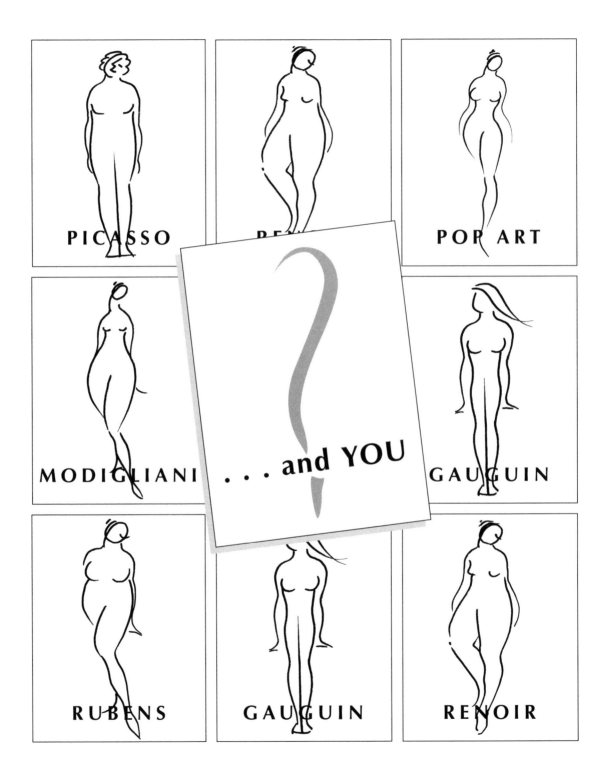

PICASSO

POP ART

MODIGLIANI

. . . and YOU

GAUGUIN

RUBENS

GAUGUIN

RENOIR

introduction

One day I went to a museum with a friend to see an exhibit of Impressionist paintings. The crowds were there early, and I had to struggle to position myself to even see a painting. Eavesdropping as I do, I heard the sighs and comments about the beauty of the women of Renoir. "Look at her. She is magnificent!" A friend leaned over to me and said, "I can't help but imagine these women throwing on their shawls after posing and walking out with confidence, knowing they were a creature of beauty."

That is when I began to notice the women looking at these works of art and saw in them what I am sure Matisse, Renoir, and Modigliani looked for in their expression of art and beauty. Different body types with angles, curves, and shapes that, while perhaps not fitting the modern "model" image, exude feminity and elegance.

We all know women who would like themselves better if they didn't have any hips or had breasts that don't have a mind of their own. But real women do have hips and breasts; women who study, take the bus, have babies, go to work, take rumba lessons, and love hot chocolate with whipped cream. Each is different, each unique. These are the real models of the master painters, and I want you to see yourself as an artist's inspiration.

Once you realize the endless variety of female beauties portrayed and loved by the great painters, you will understand why I refer to body shapes by the names of each artist or group of artists (Modigliani, Pop Art, Renoir, etc.), rather than by traditional terms, such as pear shape, hourglass, and diamond.

For example, Modigliani adored painting women with wide hips and sloping shoulders, typical of the pear shape. Renoir's delight "in the rotund architecture of shoulder, breast, hip and thigh" (Isabelle Kahn, *Renoir Nudes*) even led him to enlarge and exaggerate the body. You might be familiar with the expression "of rubenesque proportions" to describe the beauties portrayed by the artist of *Venus at the Mirror*. On the contrary, Picasso's, Henry Moore's, or Cézanne's women are rather straight; those of Monet, Balthus, or Munch may be qualified as slim; and those of Giacometti or Schiele as skinny. You will easily find hourglass types in Matisse, Lempicka, or Ingres. With their shoulders always larger than their hips, Gauguin's models evoke the typical inverted triangle shape, and some appear androgynous. In short, what really dominates here is variety.

So, whatever your shape, when standing nude in front of a mirror, you might just see yourself as a Venus stepping out of a famous painting. Hopefully, when you have gone through this book, you will not only look at a work of art but become one.

According to Michèle Didou-Manent, author of *History of the Ideal Body*, to make the body more beautiful and more attractive is "a very ancient and magical process, common to many different civilizations." As a sociocultural phenomenon, the ideal of slimness and roundness alternate throughout history. The author points out that, after the initial period of preference for roundness found in Mesopotamia, "the idea of slimness was launched on the shores of the Nile. Even the Gods and Goddesses adopted this profane stylishness." She adds, "The elegant, refined line reigned supreme for over two thousand years, up until the Roman conquest, when to please the Roman centurions, women tried to put on weight. Cleopatra probably used this stratagem." The Greeks loved slenderness, but people living in the Renaissance overwhelmingly preferred the rounder form.

Throughout the ages, people have been willing to bend to certain constraints in order to keep up with their time and sociocultural environment, as we are never indifferent as to how others judge our appearance. On the other hand, a major trend has developed in recent years toward a more and more individualistic way of dressing.

In the last fifty years, in order to become accessible to a majority of people, fashion design has evolved from an exclusive haute couture (expensive and affordable to only a minority of the population) to a more inclusive, moderate, completely ready-to-wear style. But there is a price to pay for it: From multiple fittings and adjustments to balance the shape of an individual's body, we have turned to standardization by size only, which cannot take into account the variety of body shapes.

Dressing in harmony with one's particular body shape today requires a certain effort and a certain knowledge of the subject. We'll make a comprehensive tour of it in this book. As a fashion designer and teacher, I am familiar with Parisian fashion and the specifics of the North American market. I wanted to write this book to explain to each woman, whatever age and whatever shape, how to select, match, and balance clothes and accessories to suit her.

Among the various criteria that must be taken into consideration in order to dress right, I give preeminence to shape. So don't be surprised if, in this book, I have adopted a systematic classification referring to the different body shapes. In order to dress well, you have to take your size into consideration, as well as the fact that we tend to put on weight with the years. But, whatever your size, achieving the harmonious appearance you desire will mainly depend on the way you dress according to your own body shape, which appears early in life and stays relatively constant. In other words, achieving a harmonious appearance (slimming your figure, if necessary) is first and foremost a question of overall volume *(the silhouette)*, balance, and proportion of what you wear. Furthermore, if the choice of fabrics and the color values (from dark to light) for your particular body shape are right, and if you keep details to a minimum, then you can't go wrong.

For each type of body shape, I tried to draw models with faces that recall those women that the painter loved, to better illustrate the timelessness of proposed solutions and to avoid any references to fashion trends, which are ephemeral.

How is fashion created? What *air du temps* does each creator try to capture and evoke in his collection? How does he or she interpret or misinterpret the aura of his or her time? The answer lies in what makes up life itself: art, film, music, literature, architecture, history, the news, the street. And the street? What is it? Who is it? It's you, me, and, foremost, youth, and it is through youth that future fashion trends are born. Youth implies young bodies. Does this mean that one should amalgamate the professional look of a model and looks mentioned in this book? Of course not! Just as a composer chooses the most exceptional voice or musician to interpret his work, or a country its very best athletes to defend its chances at the Olympic Games, so a fashion designer will choose a model with an exceptional body to set off a collection to advantage. The music, the lighting, the supple and airy gaits of the models, the atmosphere, the surroundings, and sometimes a touch of provocation, all contribute to the creation of modern fashion shows, which are aimed primarily at capturing media interest but also at making people dream and remember the show.

You don't need to have the body of a model in order to dress well and look great. Through numerous examples, clarified visually with illustrations, this book will give you easy-to-follow instructions. It will show you how to direct the viewer's eye to your assets and make it pass over your challenges. It will teach you the different facets that compose a harmonious, balanced look and will give you a mine of wardrobe tricks for selecting clothes that look and feel right for **your** body.

The word *"silhouette"* comes from the name *Etienne de Silhouette*, General Controller of Finance under the French King LOUIS XV. In 1759, de Silhouette created a tax to ease the burden of a century-old financial crisis. His enemies, who wanted to suggest how they look after being taxed, gave his name to cartoons representing him with only a few strokes of pencil.

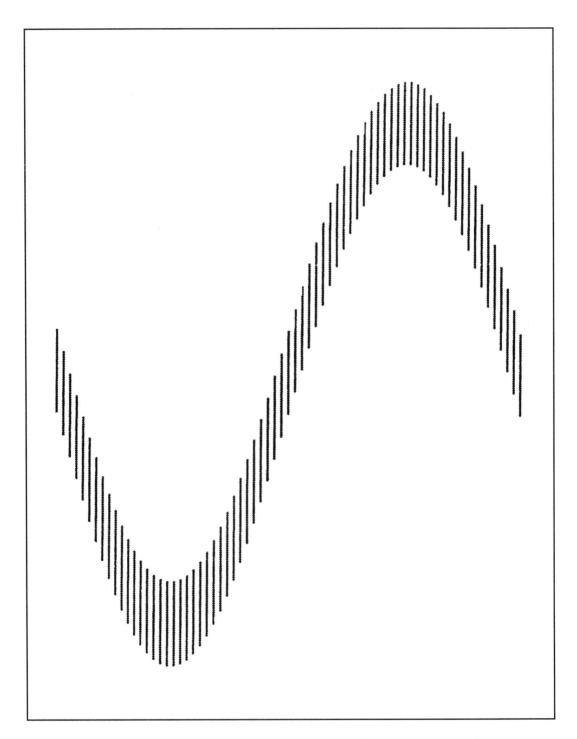

A powerful illusion: the Illusion of Day (after R.H. Day). All lines have the same length.

fundamentals

HARMONIZING SHAPE, VALUE, AND COLOR

*A*rtists, decorators, and designers have the same goal: **balance and harmony.** *They also use the same tools:* **shape, value, and color.** Just as a painter will carefully choose the surrounding colors and shapes to enhance his subject, or a decorator will thoughtfully select each subject in a room to relate them to each other or to highlight a precious piece, you can use shape, value, and color to balance and slenderize your body shape. These three elements, used wisely, will help you create, as an artist would in a painting, a perfect composition.

The primary focus is on shape and value. These are the two most powerful tools and are equal partners when it comes to slenderizing and balancing a body shape. These tools, smartly used, are the keys to successful dressing. Colors and lines are next in importance to achieve this goal.

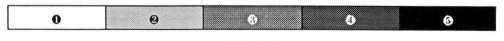

Values Scale

Values range from numbers 1, the lightest value, to 5, the darkest value. But, of course, you can have as many in-between tones as you wish.

Value 1, the white or lightest value, attracts the most attention and is therefore usually placed in such a way as to direct the viewer's eye to your assets. The lightest value is the one the eye automatically settles on first. The darker value has a receding effect, especially if you position it strategically next to the lightest value. So, with the effective placement of light, dark, and middle values, you can emphasize or downplay any body area. Once you have your value right, it is time to think about colors to get even stronger results and emotional effects.

Colors

Color Relationship and What It Can Do for You

A color's tone and value is altered when it is placed beside a different color. The selection of a desired color is not enough; you should pay close attention to the neighboring color to achieve the required effect.

- Colors can be visually moved forward or backward. Side by side, a cool color pushes a warm color forward, whereas a warm color helps a neighboring cool color to recede.

- A warm color put next to a cool color will appear even warmer and *vice versa*.

- An intense color looks even more intense beside a muted one. A dark color placed next to a light color will appear even darker. Two bright colors together will cancel each other out.

- Color can be tricky. It can even change the appearance of your complexion—make it glow or make it look drained. Never wear a color just because it is pretty. It has to flatter your skin tone.

- Your face is the center interest of your body. Frame it with a color that enhances it. Your special color or colors that flatter you most should always be placed close to your face. All the other colors in your outfit should not compete but should support this color to enhance your complexion.

- I am sure you have already heard about color coding according to your skin tone. If you don't know your colors yet, don't wait to find out. You can consult numerous good books on the subject (Mary Spillane's classic *Color Me Beautiful* or Elsa Klensch's *Style*) or take advice from an expert, such as a makeup artist, an image consultant, or an experienced salesperson in the makeup section of your department store.

Once you are acquainted with your colors and know if it is warmer or cooler shades that flatter your skin tone, cut your choices down to six or seven colors. This way, you don't need to think about mixing and matching. It's also cheaper and less time consuming. Keep two neutrals for your basic wardrobe (pants, skirts, jackets, and coats) and add some pizzazz with your accent colors for the rest of your items.

What Are Neutrals and What Are Accent Colors?

Neutral Colors

Neutrals are toned-down colors and pure black or white (achromatics), which stay **neutral** when placed side by side. For instance, because black and white and all the grays in between are neutrals, they hardly affect the appearance of a neighboring color and are therefore considered neutral. Most neutrals are a mixture of cool and warm colors; hence, they will clash neither with cool nor warm tones.

- Neutrals do not modify a strong neighboring color, but a strong neighboring color does slightly modify a neutral color. For instance, the neutral gray of a jacket seems warmer against a cool-colored shirt such as light blue or mint green, whereas a warm-colored shirt such as salmon or orange forces the gray into a cooler tone.

- Neutrals do not compete with other colors.

- Neutral colors do not cancel other colors out, but they do enhance more intensive or bright tones.

- Neutrals are easy to mix and match with most of the other colors. That is why they work so perfectly for your basic wardrobe.

As neutrals are a mixture of warm and cool colors, they can have slightly cooler or warmer hues, depending on the degree of cool or warm tones in the mixture. The hues should match your hair color and complexion.

CLASSIC NEUTRALS

WARM HUES	COOL HUES
Ivory	White
Eggshell	Ash
Beige	Smoke
Tan	Gray

Brown	Taupe
Burnt sienna	Wine
Chocolate	Charcoal
Camel	Slate
Olive	Teal
Warm umberblack (black with red or brown tones)	Blue black
	Navy

Accent Colors

An accent color is always bright or intense and best used in small quantities as a focus point to **accentuate** your assets and therefore divert attention from your challenging spots. Use it carefully. Think of it as a jewel. Bright colors surrounded with muted or neutral colors, especially teamed with black, look very luminous. An accent color can also be used as a balance strategy (large areas of neutral or muted colors can be balanced with small areas of bright colors).

Because of their brightness, accent colors are difficult to match with other strong colors. Placed side by side, they will compete with each other.

If you have a stunning figure to show off and a strong, confident personality, you can have fun with a monochromatic (one-color) outfit in a strong accent color.

ACCENT COLORS

WARM COLORS	COOL COLORS
Warm yellow	Lime green
Avocado	Turqoise
Orange	Emerald
Scarlet	Royal blue
Tangerine	Magenta
Cardinal	Fuchsia
Salmon	Shocking pink

Contrasts

Strong Contrast

Contrasts affect your skin tone as much as color does. Beware! Strong colors only suit people with dark skin tones or people with a strong color contrast between their complexion, hair, and eye color. Some people do have that striking contrast between hair, skin, and eyes, such as:

Fair skin with dark eyes and dark hair
Fair skin and fair eyes with dark hair
Blond hair with dark eyes

If you fall into this category, underline your asset with strong, intensive colors or high contrasts, such as very dark with very light tones or deep colors with bright accent colors close to your face. Muted or dull colors will make your skin look washed out. Soft blends do nothing for your complexion, either.

Soft Blends

Soft blends, such as light neutrals with white, pink with ivory, or any powder colors, flatter people with subtle contrast between their hair color, skin tone, and eye color.

Toned-down pastels or powder pastels always look more sophisticated than pure pastels. They can be mixed with each other. But avoid mixing pure pastels, please! Too cute.

Bright, intense colors, deep colors, black, or strong contrasts in clothing can be too overpowering for people with a delicate complexion and light hair. If you still want to wear black, you can soften the unwanted contrast by creating a color bridge. For instance, try a patterned scarf in black and light blue. The black in your scarf will blend into your dress, and the light blue in the scarf will complement your complexion. But you can also deemphasize a too powerful contrast with a muted-colored scarf.

Prints

Patterns can do a lot more than just look pretty. They can help balance the shape of a body, create focus points or strong optical illusions to accentuate assets or downplay challenges, and visually lengthen or widen a given shape. That's why **they affect the overall appearance of an outfit.**

Patterns should reflect your personality and underline your unique style. They can also create a color bridge between different solid-colored items. You can play with them, have fun, manipulate them, mix and match them.

The following tips and facts will help you to wisely choose the right patterns and make them work for **your** body.

- Prints should always be in scale with your size. A large-scaled pattern on a small woman looks as out of proportion as does a small-scaled pattern on a big woman.

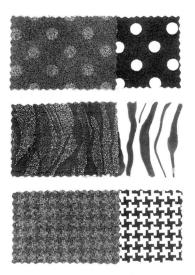

Left: Subdued color contrast.
Right: Strong color contrast.

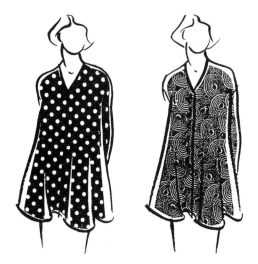

A small, widely spaced pattern with a
strong contrast *(left)* appears bolder than a
narrowly spaced print with a subdued contrast
between pattern and background *(right)*.

- Widely spaced patterns on a contrasting or light background make you look bigger, even if the pattern itself is small-scaled.

- Large-scaled prints in midtones with little value contrast don't distract as much as prints with a strong light-dark contrast.

- Eye-catching prints ask for understatement in style, as small details would be lost on a distracting pattern.

- Forget about jewelry on a loud print. It will not be noticed.

- Bold prints, just as loud colors, ask for a strong personality and a perfectly balanced figure.

- If the pattern of your clothes overwhelms your face, deemphasize the prints with a solid-colored scarf or collar.

- Don't be afraid to pair different patterns, as long as they have the same color combination. For instance, you can match blue-and-taupe checks with blue-and-taupe stripes. You can also combine two or three different flower prints with the same color palette.

- If you mix two or more different prints in the same color, make sure that one of the prints dominates to avoid boredom.

- Prints help to combine different-colored items.

- Patterns can be strategically used to draw attention to your assets and away from your challenges. For instance, if you are top-heavy but are blessed with narrow hips and shapely legs, use prints below the waistline to invite the eye down, and *vice versa*. Try a patterned top to bring the eye up if you are bottom-heavy.

- Use large-scaled stripes, large plaids, or geometric prints for loosely fitting styles only.

- Large plaids are more slimming when cut on the bias.

- Make sure that plaids or horizontal stripes match at seams. An interrupted pattern is a telltale sign of poor craftsmanship.

- Select prints that are appropriate for the occasion and your lifestyle.

- Clothes in extremely trendy patterns are outdated quickly. Garments with an outdated print are difficult to update with other items.

- Classic prints never go out of style. Choose houndstooth, pinstripes, checks, glen plaids, chevrons, and herringbone for a sporty look or paisleys, pin dots, polka dots, medallion, foulard, or classic florals for a more feminine look.

- Don't let yourself be used as a human billboard for a clothing label or any other brand name. The big lettering emblazoned across your chest or back are seldom in scale with your body and are usually badly placed on the clothing itself.

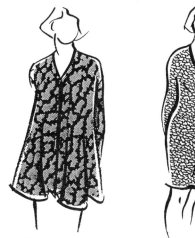

Here again, large-scaled prints *(left)* look best on generously cut styles in a drapey fabric. For body-fitted styles in knit *(right)*, use small- or medium-scaled all-over prints which tend to camouflage any possible little bulge.

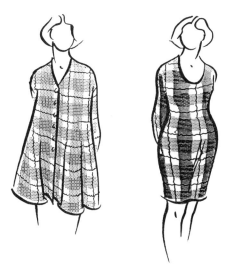

Large-scaled plaids can look terrific on big women, but in loosely fitted styles only *(left)*. Plaids and stripes in a body-hugging style *(right)* can be very unflattering, as they emphasize curves and therefore make one look bigger.

Fabrics

It is the fiber content, the yarn structure, the type of weave or knit, and the finish that will give a fabric a specific appearance. Each of these four elements affects the look, the drape, the weight, and the quality of the fabric. Fabric can be heavy or light, rough or smooth, warm or cool, soft or coarse, thin or thick, lustrous or matte, opaque or transparent, fluid or crisp. It can shape a body, drape around a body, cling to a body, stand away from a body, or fall straight. Whatever the style, it is the weight and the drape of a fabric that determine the shape of a garment; **therefore, always choose a fabric that lends itself to a given silhouette.**

For instance, an A-line or a flared skirt in a stiff fabric tends to stand away from the body, whereas the same style in a soft, drapable fabric provides a narrow, streamlined silhouette. An oversized, unstructured jacket in a stiff, bulky fabric will make you look big, whereas the same style in a soft, drapable fabric will slenderize a body.

Weaves are usually stronger than knits. They retain pleats, creases, and the form of a garment better, but are less flexible and therefore need more darts and seams for a perfect fit. Tight weaves, such as denim or corduroy, are stiff and bulky and should be avoided over the less flattering parts of your body. Loose weaves, such as gauze, voile, chiffon, or challis, are drapy and are more appropriate for loose-fitting, gathered, or drapy styles, whereas firm, medium-weight fabrics are better suited for angular or semifitted styles.

Knits are soft, flexible, stretchy, drapable, and are great for loosely fitted, generously sized styles, as they provide an excellent drape. They are also perfect for semifitted or body-contoured styles (for a

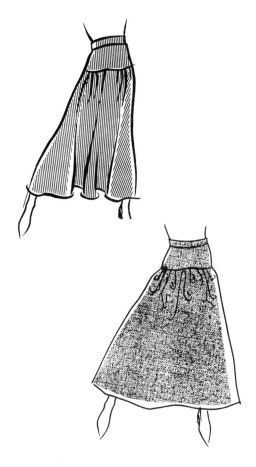

Both skirts have the same style. The skirt on the left is cut out of a drapey, soft fabric, which gives it a streamlined, slenderizing silhouette; the skirt on the right is made out of a stiff fabric, which stands away from the body and makes you appear much bigger than you actually are.

perfectly balanced figure only!), as they stretch easily over curves. Fitted styles in knits tend to bag or sag unless they come with a small percentage of stretch fibers such as spandex or Lycra. Garments with these blends don't lose their initial form as quickly as knits without these fibers. With pure wool or cotton knits, make sure that skirts and pants are lined at the largest area of your body or where there is the biggest pull on the garment, such as the knees or the behind.

Select fabrics from natural fibers for clothes worn close to your skin. Natural fibers such as wool or silk come from animals, and linen, nettle, cotton, hemp, or ramie, from plants. Natural fibers absorb body moisture, let your skin breathe, are easy to care for, have longevity, and never look cheap.

Blends are a mixture of natural and synthetic fibers. In a good-quality blend, the content of the synthetic fiber should not exceed 25 percent. Fabrics of both types of fibers combined adapt well to our lifestyle. These blends look and feel natural, are absorbent, easy to care for, and don't wrinkle.

For outerwear, don't ignore the 100 percent man-made fabrics. Polyester or microfibers don't look cheap anymore. They can have the look and touch of a natural fabric and are light, soft, and fluid. Parkas, for instance, don't need to be bulky and heavy. Made out of these new, innovative fabrics, they can compete in warmth and comfort with any traditional parka but are lighter and easier to care for.

There are some man-made fabrics you should avoid such as acrylics and orlon. They are not absorbent, and they build up static electricity and therefore tend to cling.

More Tips

- Garments in quality fabrics maintain their initial form, and they drape well.

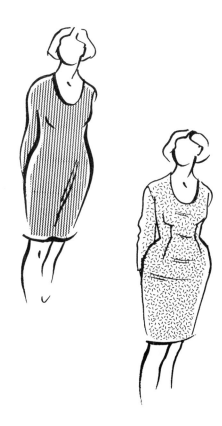

Top: A well-proportioned body can be enhanced with a curve-hugging dress in a soft knit.
Bottom: A stiff fabric is not appropriate for a tightly fitted style. It creates horizontal wrinkles, so it won't give the desired streamlined look, and it makes even a dream figure appear large.

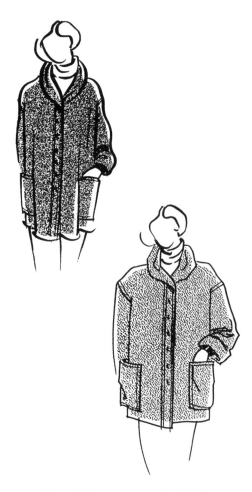

Two different fabrics give a completely different shape to the jackets. The jacket on the *top* is made of a soft, drapey fabric, which gives it a narrow, streamlined silhouette; the same style made out of a bulky or stiff fabric, as is the one on the *bottom,* will make you appear bigger than you are.

- Always wear a slip or camisole under a clingy fabric.

- When mixing two different textures for a layered look, keep the top layer slightly heavier.

- Combine differently textured surfaces, such as matte with shiny or rough with smooth, to add interest to a monochromatic outfit.

- Heavy, bulky textures will swamp a small woman.

- Shiny fabrics make you look bigger, and matte fabrics have a receding effect.

- Loosely fitted styles, body-contoured styles, or layered looks demand soft, drapable fabrics, whereas tailored styles ask for a firm texture.

- Oversized styles in soft, drapable, nonclingy fabrics can make you look smaller, whereas oversized styles in bulky, heavy fabrics always make you look bigger.

- Look for clothes in fabrics you can wear all year round.

- Always read the care label on a garment so that you know how to care for it.

- Clothes in quality fabrics look luxurious, whereas clothes in poor-quality fabrics always look cheap.

- Stretchy textures softly hug curves, but beware: curves are beautiful, bulges are ugly.

OPTICAL ILLUSIONS AS APPLIED TO FASHION

Sometimes we don't see a line, a surface, a detail, or a color exactly as it actually is but quite differently due to an optical illusion. In fashion, we could use those effects to give a new silhouette to a particular shape by either enhancing its assets or disguising its challenges or both.

Below are the most useful of these optical illusions.

Illusions Affecting the Way We See Lines

Vertical-Horizontal Effect

Generally, vertical lines or stripes lengthen, horizontal ones widen. This is because a line is first seen in the direction of its length.

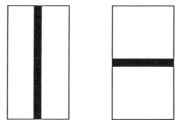

Both rectangles are the same size, but the one with the vertical line *(left)* seems longer than the one with the horizontal line *(right)*, as one line, or very few lines, will invite the eye in a given direction.

In some cases, however, horizontal stripes can lengthen and therefore make you look slimmer.

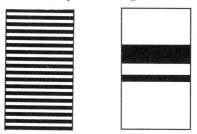

Regular, narrow spacing between thin horizontal lines *(left)* do not widen as the eye is led up and down, which therefore has a lengthening effect. Irregular spacing or large horizontal lines *(right)* invite the eye to look across and thus seems wider.

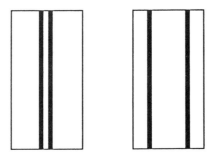

Narrow, vertical lines *(left)* invite the eye up and down at the center and therefore elongate. (Think of a jacket worn open, a centerfront piping, or an oblong scarf worn vertically.) Widely spaced vertical lines *(right)* will lead the eye outward and will make you look broader (a double-breasted jacket with widely spaced buttons or a wide front panel, for instance).

The Angle Effect

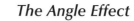
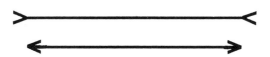

A line ending with angles turned inward *(bottom)* appears shorter than a line ending with angles turned outward *(top)*, though both have the same length. The first type of angle invites the eye outside and therefore lengthens, while the second has a shortening effect.

The Split Effect

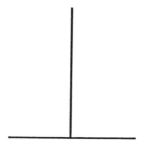

The vertical line seems longer than the horizontal one of equal size. Generally, a line split in half appears shorter, as does the horizontal one above.

The Diagonal Effect

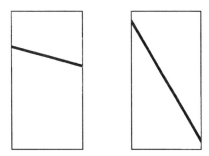

The steeper the diagonal, the narrower a rectangle seems.

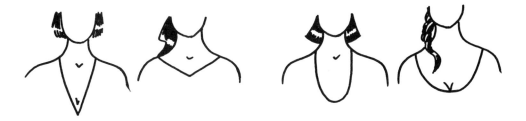

For example, the steeper the diagonal of a V neck, the more slimming it is *(left)*. The same principle applies to curves. The deeper a curve is, the more slenderizing it is *(right)*.

Illusions Affecting the Way We See Surfaces

Horizontal Divisions

  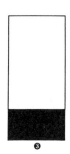 

(1) Monochromatic, unbroken space lengthens the most.
(2) Horizontally divided space of equal size appears widest because it leads the eye across.
(3) and (4) Extremely unequally divided space lengthens as well, because it invites the eye up and down. (Think of a jacket paired with a mini or a long dress teamed with a cropped top.)

Influence of the Background

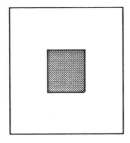 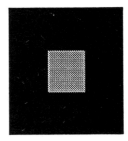

Identical values can appear different with different backgrounds.

Both gray center squares have identical values. But the gray of the center square *on the left* seems darker against a lighter background, whereas the dark background of the square *on the right* forces the gray into a lighter value.

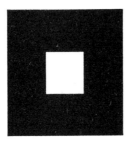 

A light surface on a dark background advances, appearing to jump off the dark background, and it looks bigger than a dark surface of equal size on a light background. The dark square *(right)* recedes and looks smaller. The white square *(left)* captures the eye first and therefore dominates over the dark one.

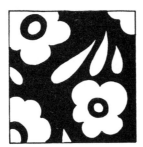 

The same goes for prints. A light pattern on a dark background *(left)* appears bigger and more powerful than a dark pattern of equal size on a light background *(right)*.

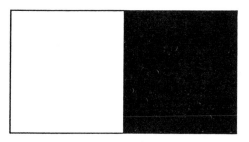

Placed side by side, light values appear bigger than reality, whereas dark values appear smaller than reality. The light square seems bigger than the black one of the same size.

General Illusions

Size-Contrast Factor

Lines, surfaces, volumes, details, and prints all appear larger than they are if contrasted with things smaller, and *vice versa*.

Tight-Fitting or Loose-Fitting Effect

A tight garment or part of a garment reveals the real forms of the body, while loose or over-sized clothes disguise the exact shape. The first is used to emphasize assets and the second to counter challenges.

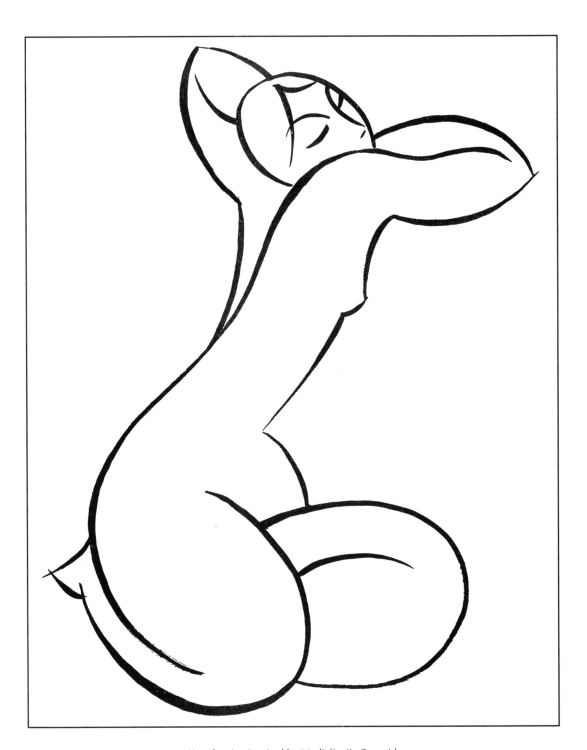

Line drawing inspired by Modigliani's *Caryatid*.

modigliani

Amedeo Modigliani (1884–1920)

Born in Livorno, Italy, to a French mother and an Italian father, the young Modigliani came to Paris in 1906, at the age of twenty-two, where he lived a true bohemian life till his death at thirty-six.

Paris was then the capital city of the European avant-garde. Modigliani, or "Modi" (allusion to *peintre maudit*, or "accursed painter"), met Matisse, Picasso, and the poet Jean Cocteau, but his best friends were probably the French painter Maurice Utrillo and the Romanian sculptor Constantin Brancusi.

Modigliani loved women and captured their beauty by painting his subjects with delicate torsos, sloping, narrow shoulders, and wide hips and thighs. This is especially evident in his paintings of Jeanne Hébuterne, his last companion. Her wistful elegance graces his canvases and exudes beyond the frame. Usually referred to as a pear-shaped figure, I now call this the Modigliani shape.

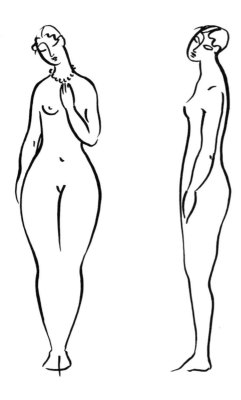

CHARACTERISTICS

1. Slender neck

2. *Narrow shoulders (often sloping)*

3. *Small bust*

4. Refined rib cage

5. Shapely waist

6. *Generous lower hips*

7. *Full thighs*

Modigliani Shape

To Enhance and Balance Your Silhouette

Focus attention to the upper part of your body.

■

Enlarge your shoulder area to balance wider hips.

■

Suggest, without emphasizing, your fine waist and midriff.

■

Downplay your lower torso.

Modigliani (Pear) Shape
General Recommendations

SHAPES AND SILHOUETTES	**Skirts and Pants**	<ul><li>Beware of too-tight skirts. While you'll want to show off your shapely waist, such skirts will focus attention on your bottom. Your skirts and pants must fit loosely around the hips and thighs, even if it means that you have to alter the waistband to fit you.</li><li>Straight skirts in crisp fabric should be tapered toward the hemline to avoid a heavy, square look.</li><li>A-line skirts must be made of soft, flowing fabrics to create a narrow silhouette (for details see "Fabrics" on page 25).</li><li>Knife pleats worn with a top long enough to cover your bottom would also provide a streamlined silhouette.</li><li>Pants should be made out of soft, flowing fabric only. Select styles with open tucks or elastic at the waist and wide enough to drape loosely around your hips. Have them slightly tapered from the broadest part of your bottom down to the hemline.</li></ul>
	Tops and Dresses	<ul><li>Always, always wear shoulder pads!</li><li>Your best buys are semifitted or tailored tops to accentuate your fine waist and bustline. Wear them high-waisted to help lengthen and slim your bottom half.</li><li>The hemline of a top should end below your buttock for medium to tall women or just above the hipbone if you are short.</li></ul>

SHAPES AND SILHOUETTES (Continued)	**Tops and Dresses** (Continued)	• Avoid tops that end at the broadest part of your bottom. You don't want to expose your challenges! • With your delicate top and broad bottom, it might prove difficult to find a good-fitting dress. Consider having one tailored. • The best style for your body shape is an empire dress. This style fits snugly over the bustline and softly flares out. This will hint at, but not emphasize, your shapely middle and at the same time will not reveal your generous hips and thighs. • For dresses, use drapy fabrics only. Layers at the top will also help to balance your ample bottom half.
COLORS AND PRINTS	**Skirts and Pants**	• Keep colors dark, neutral, or muted. These shades help to downplay your challenges. • With such a wonderfully feminine body shape, choose old-fashioned, delicate, feminine prints or fine, small prints. Contrasting or loud colors will only attract unwanted attention to the lower part of your body.
	Tops and Dresses	• Feel free to experiment with colors as long as they suit your personality or mood. The choices are endless, as long as you focus attention on your slender top. Choose colors that flatter your facial skin tone. • Select feminine prints, such as florals, polka dots, gingham check, paisley, pin dots, or soft, delicate abstracts.

FABRICS	**Skirts and Pants**	• Choose firm fabrics for straight-lined, tapered skirts to counter your curves, or look for fabrics that are soft, fluid, and drape well, such as medium-weight knits, jersey, fluid polyester fibers, washed silk, crepe, chiffon, challis, viscose, and rayon for slightly gathered or flared skirts.
	Tops and Dresses	• For daytime wear, select tight or firm weaves, such as gabardine or linen. For evening, wear taffetas, raw silk, tapestries, and brocade for your semifitted or straight-lined tops, and fluid fabrics for your dresses. With your delicate torso, here you can afford some extra textures. Have some fun with fake furs, mohair, quilts, or fluffy fabrics.
DETAILS	**Skirts and Pants**	• Avoid horizontal seams, piping, edging, trims, and yokes. You do not need any eye-catching details in that area. Patch pockets, bows, ruffles, and ties will only add additional bulk where you don't want it and emphasize your broader bottom. Steer clear of any appliqué at hem level, as this would invite the eye down, make you look shorter, and give an unbalanced appearance to your shape.
	Tops and Dresses	• Wide-open necklines, cowls, boat necks, and shoulder yokes all create horizontal lines that help the eye move across the shoulder area. This gives a widening effect, which balances your heavier hips. • Contrasting-colored or shiny buttons, ruffles, bows, ribbons, trimmings, appliqués, breast pockets, and interesting textures all bring the eye up and draw attention away from your bottom half. Just don't overdo it! Stick to one or two eye-catching details. The simpler a garment, the more refined and expensive it looks.

ACCESSORIES	Shoes	<ul><li>Go for low-cut, oval openings to visually lengthen your legs.</li><li>Avoid horizontal lines such as T or ankle straps.</li><li>Beware of heavy buckles and bows on all footwear as well as heavy, chunky boots.</li><li>Choose hosiery, shoes, and skirts in the same tone value.</li><li>Avoid heavy, square, flat heels. A 1½" or 2" (3–5 cm) heel, depending on your outfit, will be more flattering to you than a flat heel.</li></ul>
	Handbags	<ul><li>Large, bulky, overstuffed bags do not flatter your figure.</li><li>Try to wear your shoulder bag above the hip area. This will eliminate additional bulk around your hips and thighs.</li><li>At work, a smart tote, soft and medium-sized, works well for you.</li><li>For a dressier look, choose a medium- to a small-sized handbag or a clutch purse. This complements and suits your feminine figure.</li></ul>
	Belts	<ul><li>Yes! Do wear belts for your shapely waist; but, as you probably want to move the eye to your middle, away from your bottom, consider wearing an open jacket or cardigan over pants and skirts.</li></ul>

ACCESSORIES (Continued)	Scarves	▪ Wear scarves and shawls horizontally or diagonally draped. You can keep them in place with a brooch or a hidden safety pin at the shoulder. Don't hide your slender neck; play with colors to bring the eye up.
	Jewelry	▪ Use necklaces, earrings, and brooches to focus attention on your face. Wear your necklaces short and your brooches close to the shoulder area. ▪ For earrings, choose small studs, hoops, and drops to go with your long neck. ▪ Delicate jewelry: antique jewelry; pearls; filigree; and precious, refined designs will really suit your feminine type better than modern, large, overpowering pieces.

TIP: Wear a short silk camisole under a long top, but wear it over your pants or skirt. Yes, over! This way, your tunic won't cling to your bottom garments. Your outfit will look much more chic. This trick is especially recommended for fine synthetic knits, which tend to cling.

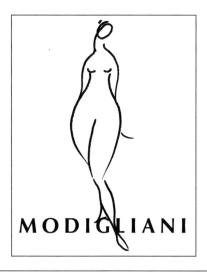

MODIGLIANI

Empire-Line

The Most Flattering Silhouette for the Modigliani Shape

This style also enhances the Renoir shape.

■

1. A lace choker leads the eye to your slender neck.

2. A boat neck visually widens narrow shoulders.

3. A caped kimono (with shoulder pads) extends your shoulders to balance your broader hips.

4. A fitted bust accentuates your delicate upper torso.

5. A slightly flared skirt gives room to generous thighs.

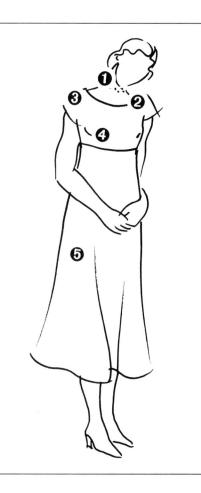

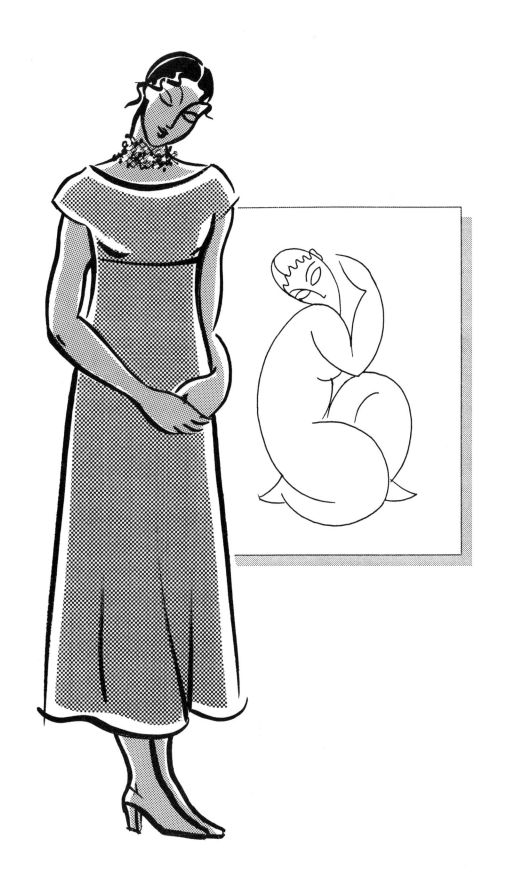

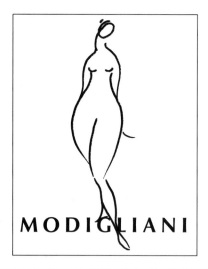

MODIGLIANI

Semifitted Three-Quarters-Length Jacket Paired with a Short Skirt

A Stylish Combination for the Modigliani Shape

■

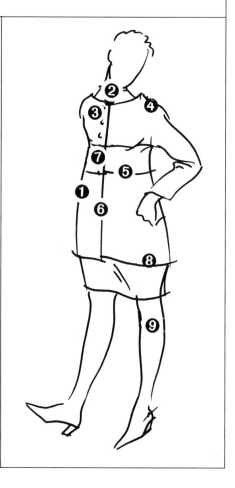

1. The straight lines of the high-waisted, semifitted jacket, cut in a firm fabric, counters voluptuous thighs and makes you appear slimmer.

2. A choker draws attention to your slender neck.

3. A lighter value at shoulder area widens and helps the eye settle on your upper torso first.

4. Set-in sleeves with square shoulder pads straighten round, narrow shoulders.

5. A waist seam slightly above your natural waistline elongates the lower torso.

6. Invisible buttons below the waistline help to downplay that area.

7. Wide, horizontal stripes lead the eye across your shapely midriff and waist.

8. A three-quarters-length jacket covers your generous hips. The short skirt tapers toward the hemline to avoid a square, boxy look.

9. The same tone value from waist to toe visually lenghtens your legs.

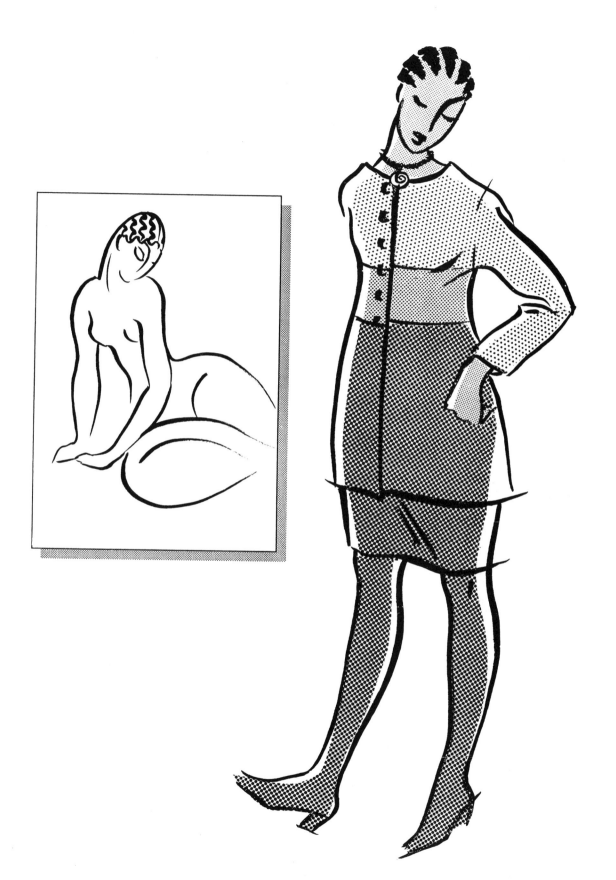

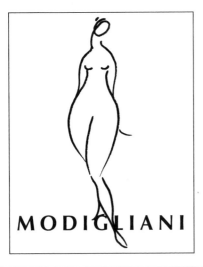

MODIGLIANI

A Semifitted, Hipbone-Length Top

A Flattering Length If Paired with a Deeper-Toned Skirt

■

1. A wide, ribbed cowl provides a textural contrast to draw attention to your neck and to widen your shoulder area.

2. Short sleeves balance generous thighs.

3. A semifitted top suggests a shapely waist without emphasizing curvacious hips.

4. A strong color contrast between top and bottom items creates a horizontal line **above** hip level and helps the eye pass over your hips and thighs.

5. Open darts give room to voluptuous thighs.

6. Top-stitched center-front seam elongates your lower torso.

7. The skirt is tapered toward the hem for a narrow silhouette.

8. Hosiery that is tone-in-tone with the skirt elongates legs.

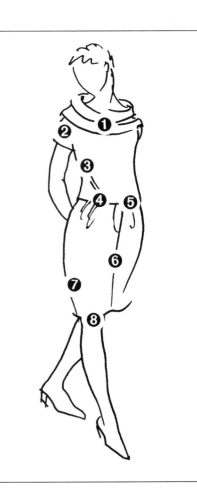

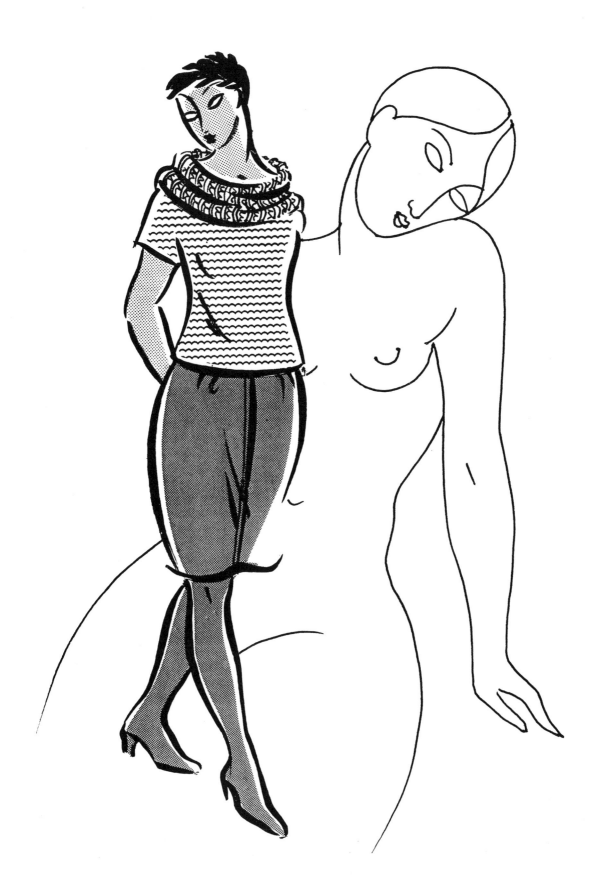

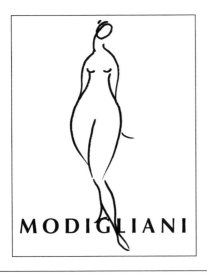

MODIGLIANI

A Maxi Vest

Provides an Elongating Silhouette for the Modigliani Shape

This vest also flatters the Renoir shape.

■

1. A colorful scarf draws attention to your top.

2. The armhole of the vest extends your shoulder bone, which widens narrow shoulders (can be taken one size up).

3. The sleeve of a brightly colored bodice maximizes narrow shoulders.

4. A cinched waist (under an open top layer only) reveals your slender waist.

5. Loosely fitting pants (in a soft, drapable fabric only) provide a streamlined look and allow for more ease at the hip area.

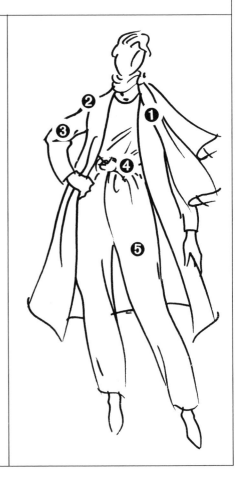

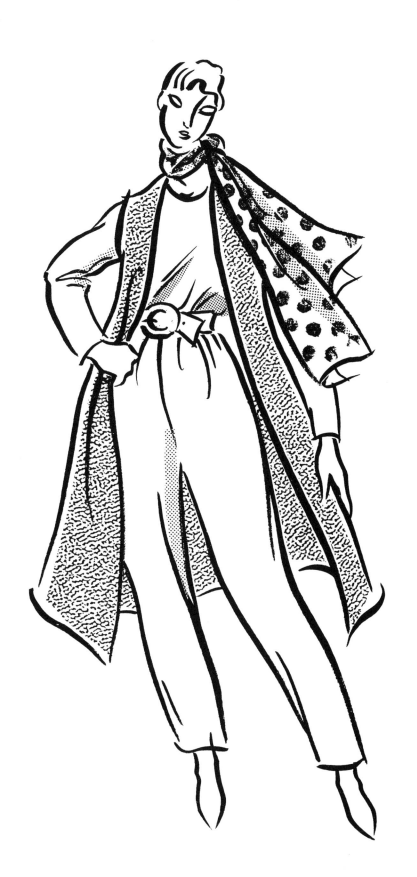

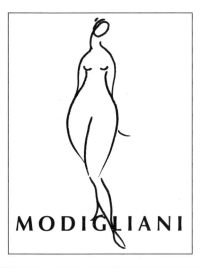

MODIGLIANI

A Cropped Top with a Wrap Skirt

An Ideal Silhouette for the Modigliani Shape

■

1. A boat neck and cape kimono trimmed with a wide border widens your shoulder area.

2. The cropped top, also trimmed with a wide border, invites the eye across a delicate midriff, reveals a fine waist, and balances generous hips.

3. Wrap skirt (in soft fabric only) gives ease at the hip area.

NOTE: *Remember! Long compared to short seems even longer. The cropped top gives the illusion of a longer bottom in proportion.*

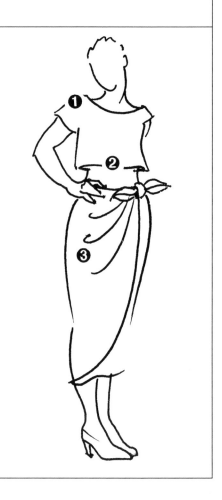

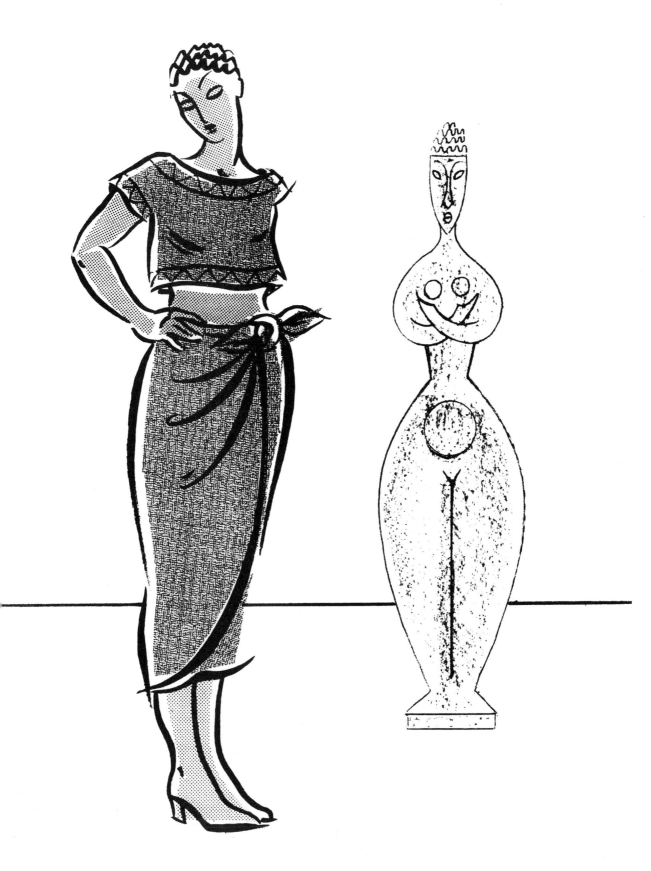

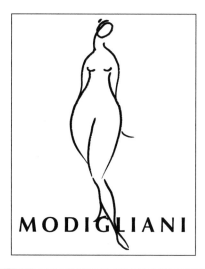

MODIGLIANI

Long, Semifitted Dress (Slightly A-Lined) Topped with a Bolero Jacket

A Winner for the Modigliani Shape

This silhouette also flatters the Renoir shape.

■

1. Drop earrings flatter a slender neck.

2. The braid-trimmed and beaded bolero jacket definitely catches the eye and draws attention to above the waist.

3. The dress is slightly A-lined to give ease at the hip area.

4. Black, the most receding color, plays down your curved hips and thighs, especially if teamed with a lighter top.

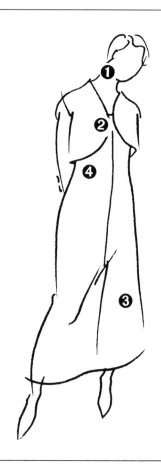

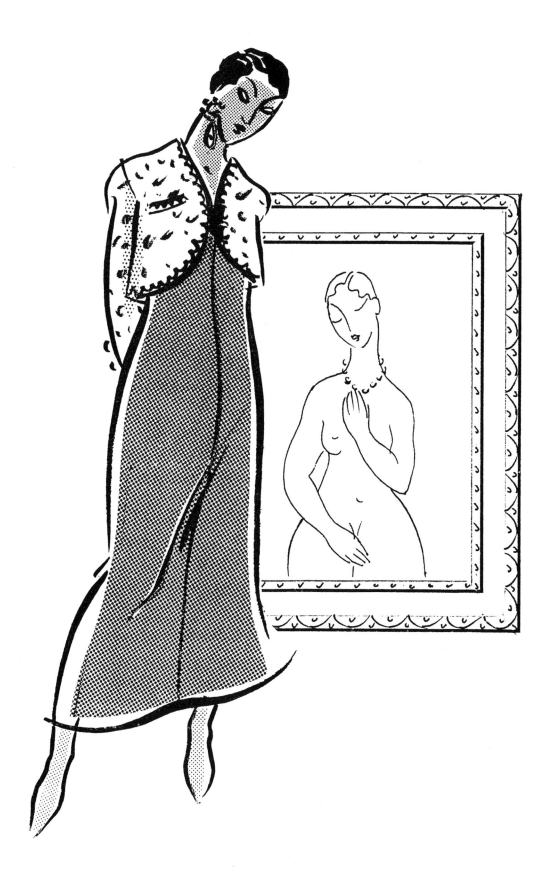

SUMMARY:

Silhouettes that flatter the Modigliani shape minimize your figure challenges and show off your assets so you will look slimmer.

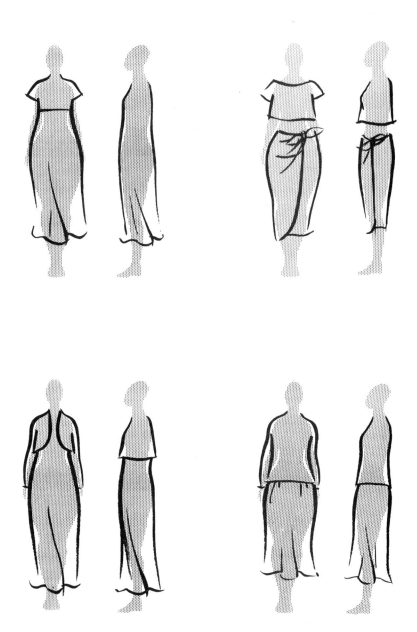

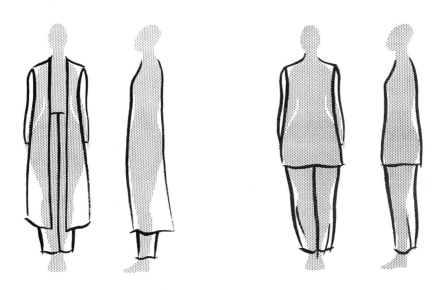

Silhouettes that hide your assets or expose your figure challenges make you look bigger.

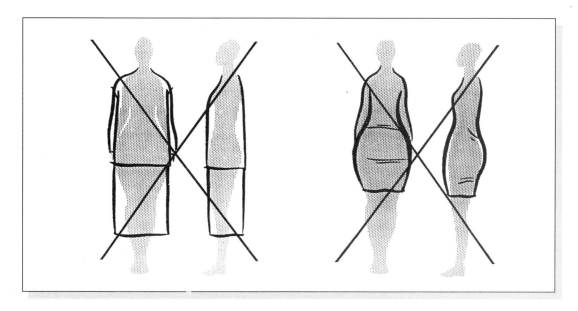

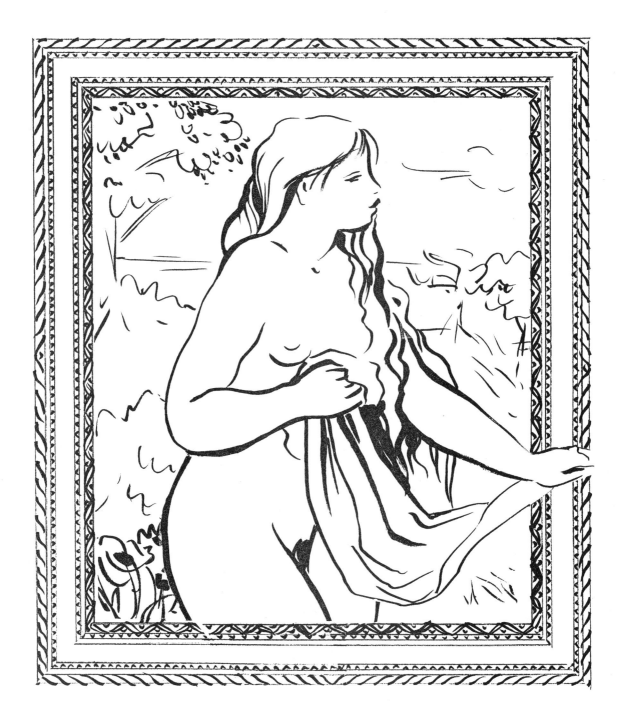

Line drawing inspired by Renoir's painting *Bather with Long Hair.*

renoir

Auguste Renoir (1841–1919)

Born in the Southwest of France to a poor family (his father was a tailor, his mother a seamstress), Auguste Renoir (or Pierre-Auguste, as he is known in America) came to Paris at an early age.

He started to work as a porcelain painter, spending a lot of time at the Louvre, then entered the Ecole des Beaux-Arts and became a friend of Monet. He lived on the slopes of Montmartre, and his life, unlike many artists, revolved around his family. Auguste Renoir's paintings often evoke family harmony and *joie de vivre*.

His nudes have been compared to flowers, voluptuous and delicate at the same time, and always larger at the bottom. Evident in his paintings is the ease, comfort, and delight that his models took in their bodies. The eye is drawn to their lightness and the carefree manner in which they carry themselves. Known traditionally as a diamond shape, I refer to this form as the Renoir. You may identify yourself in one of his paintings. If so, be like Berthe, Nini, or Aline, his favorite models: happy, relaxed, confident, and at home in the sensuousness of your body.

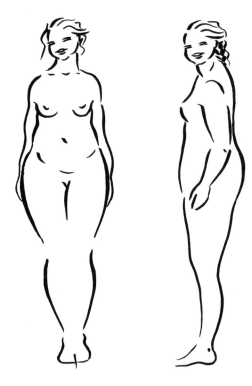

CHARACTERISTICS

1. Narrow shoulders

2. Small bust

3. Full waist

4. **Broad hips**

5. **Generous thighs**

Renoir Shape

———

To Balance and Slenderize Your Silhouette

Create a focal point above your waist.

■

Broaden your shoulder area to counter your bottom half.

■

Divert attention from your lower region.

———

Renoir (Diamond) Shape
General Recommendations

SHAPES AND SILHOUETTES	**Skirts and Pants**	<ul><li>Wear skirts and pants straight, slightly tapered in toward the hemline, and elasticized at the waist for a comfortable fit and for ease at the middle, hips, and thighs.</li><li>Skirts and pants in knits without a waistband at all are the most comfortable.</li><li>As your thighs and knees are not your best assets, make sure to cover them. Beware of maxi-length (ankle-length), as this would make you look shorter and heavier.</li><li>Pants should be straight, gently tapered toward the hem, in soft, drapable fabrics for a narrow silhouette.</li><li>Beware of too much width at the hemline, such as palazzo pants, bell-bottoms, or wide, straight trousers. Those silhouettes weigh you down, visually shorten your legs, and make you look bottom-heavy.</li></ul>
	Tops and Dresses	<ul><li>As your shoulders are narrower than your bottom, do wear shoulder pads for a more balanced look. However, they do not need to be too large, especially if you are short.</li><li>Set-in sleeves are a good choice for you, as they straighten your round shoulders, but make sure the armhole is deep enough to accommodate your full arms.</li><li>Tops should be fitted over your bust and then flare out toward middle hips and thighs.</li></ul>

SHAPES AND SILHOUETTES (Continued)	**Tops and Dresses** (Continued)	• Wear your jackets loose, unstructured, and long to cover your bottom and thighs. Make sure they are large enough and don't pull at the broadest part of your bottom. • Buy your tops and dresses a size bigger and have them fitted at bust level. • Your best silhouettes for dresses are empire styles, trapeze, tent dresses, and tunics that are slightly flared, all shapes that fit over your bust but disguise your middle, hips, bottom, and thighs (in drapable fabrics only).
COLORS AND PRINTS	**Skirts and Pants**	• Your best buys are neutral, subdued, or dark values for skirts and pants. • Your prints should be medium to large in scale, tone-in-tone, with soft, muted flower prints or abstracts. Geometric prints or angular lines do not suit your feminine figure. • Loud, contrasting colors and big or widely spaced patterns will accent your challenges, and very small patterns will not suit your build.
	Tops and Dresses	• Do use colors for your tops. Choose the ones that are most flattering to your facial skin tone. Big women are usually blessed with a lovely complexion.

FABRICS		• For generously cut styles, fabrics should be soft and fluid, such as voile, chiffon, seersucker, georgette, knits, jerseys, crepes, microfibers, washed silk, soft flannels, gabardine, knit velvet, and challis, so they can drape nicely around your body. • For an open, straight-lined top layer, you can opt for a slightly firmer fabric. • For fine, transparent, or clingy fabrics, a nonclingy camisole underneath is a must. • Stretch fibers, such as Lycra, spandex, or blends, should be worn under a loose top only. • Medium-weight jersey and knits will be the best for you. • Steer clear of stiff fabrics, such as denim, heavy cottons, corduroy, taffeta, burlap, raw silk, or any bulky fabrics, such as quilts, fur, mohair, or heavy tweeds.
DETAILS	**Skirts and Pants**	• Avoid patch pockets, horizontal edging, trimmings, ruffles, and appliqués, so as not to draw attention to that area.
	Tops and Dresses	• Breast pockets, cowl necks, boat necks, bertha collars, and shoulder yokes widen your shoulder area. • Beware of dainty details. They will look lost on you and make you look bigger in proportion.

ACCESSORIES	Shoes	• Oval, low-cut shoes, if high on the side, will create a narrow opening. The opening of your shoe frames the instep of your foot in a way similar to a décolleté neckline. Remember: Long, narrow openings slenderize; horizontal lines or wide openings enlarge. • T-straps would divide your foot in half and visually shorten your legs. • If your legs are on the heavy side, go for sheer or semi-opaque hosiery, and match them with your shoes and skirts by keeping them in the same tone value. • A medium-high heel, 1½"–2½" (3.8–6.4 cm) depending on your outfit, will look best on you. • Spiked heels or heels that are too heavy or chunky might throw you out of proportion.
	Handbags	• Avoid bulky bags. Keep them flat and medium-sized. • Very sporty or very angular designs will not fit your feminine figure. • Wear your shoulder bag short, so it falls above hip level, to avoid drawing attention to your hips. • Keep your bags neutral, and save the eye-catching colors for accessories close to your face.
	Belts	• None

ACCESSORIES (Continued)	**Scarves**	▪ Have fun with scarves. They are your most important accessory to finish off your outfit. ▪ Play with colors to give your wardrobe a lift and to draw attention above the waist. ▪ Wear them loose around your neck. ▪ Choose soft, drapable, loose weaves or transparent scarves, which don't create too much bulk and hide your feminine décolleté. ▪ Shawls, horizontally or diagonally draped, bring the eye up and let it travel across your shoulders to balance your broader bottom half.
	Jewelry	▪ Earrings, brooches, or necklaces brighten up your face, add sparkle to your outfit, and divert attention from the broader part of your body. ▪ Wear your necklaces or brooches above bust level. ▪ Avoid pendants, as they would lead the eye to your larger middle. ▪ The best length for your necklaces is just below the collarbone. ▪ Consider your size and type when buying jewelry. Choose costume jewelry or classic styles as long as they are not too tiny.

TIP: Flowing loosely fitted skirts or pants are best lined so that they won't cling to your thighs as you move.

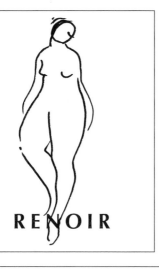

R E N O I R

Empire Dress

A Swinging, No-Waist Silhouette to Enhance the Renoir Shape

*This style also enhances
the Modigliani shape.*

■

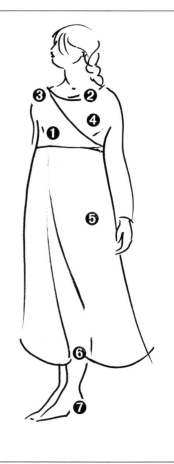

1. Fitted over the bust, this style does not swamp your upper torso.

2. The wide neckline leads the eye across the shoulder area.

3. Small shoulder pads balance voluptuous hips and thighs.

4. The textural contrast between rough and smooth at the bust area brings the eye up.

5. A slightly flared skirt gives thighs extra room.

6. Hose and shoes are toned in with the dress to give an elongating look.

7. A medium to high heel works best with this silhouette.

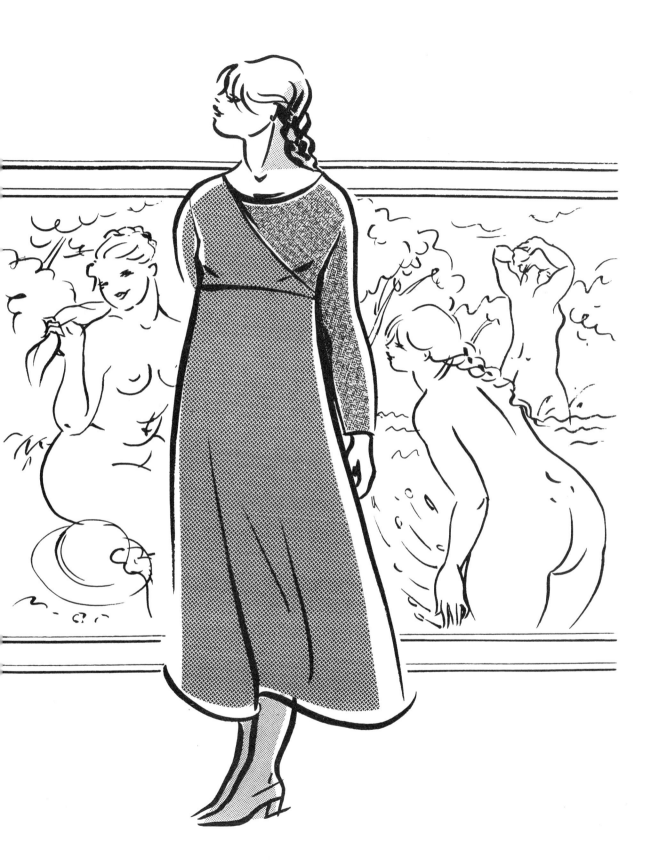

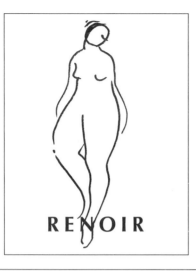

RENOIR

Long Vest Flared Toward Hips and Thighs with Fluid, Tapered Pants

A Silhouette That Flatters the Renoir Shape

This style also suits the Modigliani shape.

■

1. The bodice in a lighter or vivid color creates a focal point close to your face and visually widens your shoulder area.

2. A brooch just below your shoulder invites the eye outward and broadens your shoulders.

3. Armholes placed one inch outside the shoulder bones give the illusion of wider shoulders to balance a broader lower torso and thighs.

4. Fitted over the bust and then softly flared toward the hemline, this style does not hide your delicate bust and gives ease to hips and thighs.

5. Side slits in a long, vertical curve give additional room for a generous bottom.

6. Matching, loose-fitting pants tapered toward the hemline give an unbroken, streamlined silhouette.

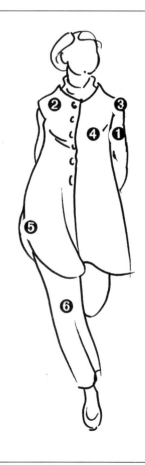

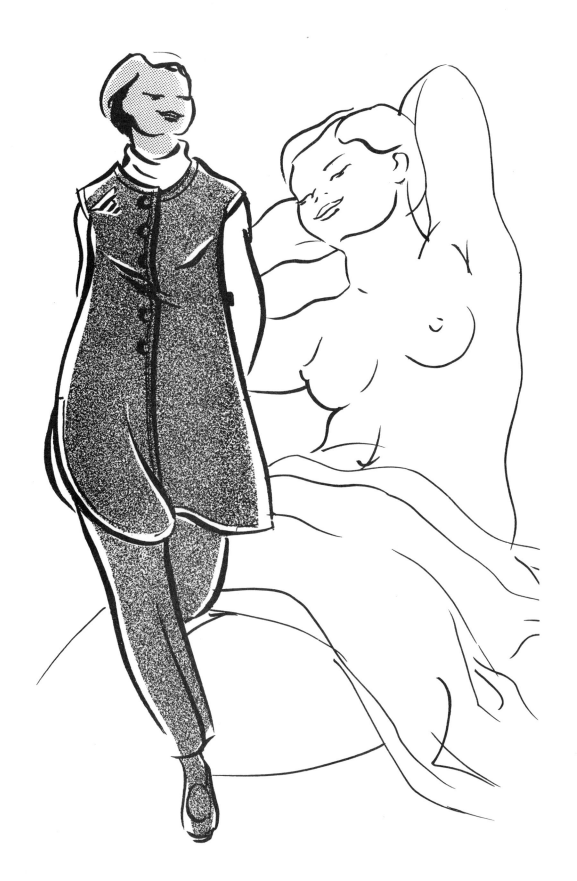

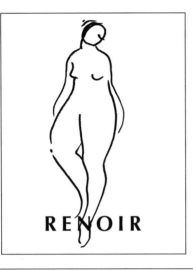

RENOIR

Duster-Length Vest

For a Streamlined, Lengthening Silhouette

A long, unbuttoned vest suits all body shapes.

■

1. A deeply colored vest over a contrasting, light-colored top invites the eye to your top and visually widens your shoulder area to balance your generous bottom half.

2. A long side slit gives ease at hips and thighs.

3. A deeply colored skirt helps the eye pass over your challenges.

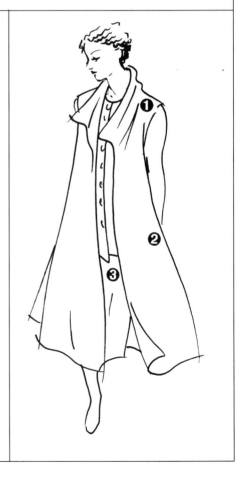

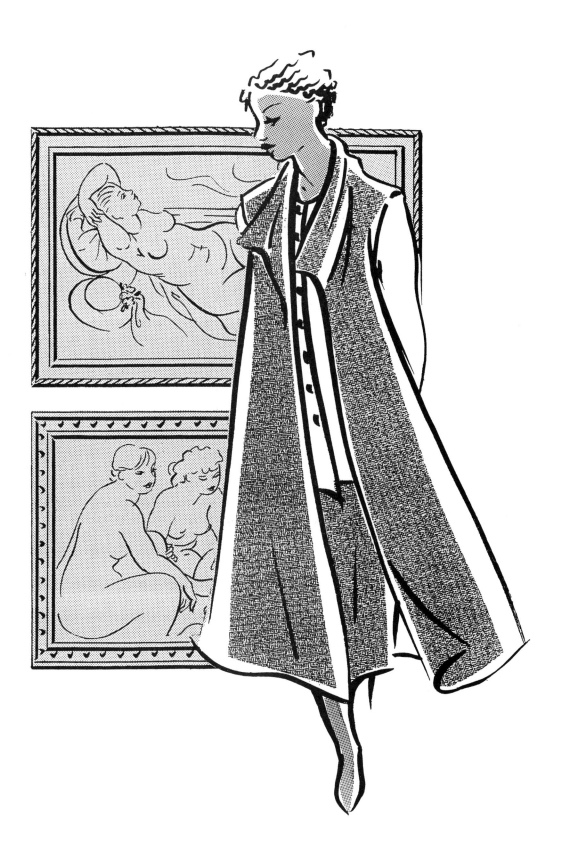

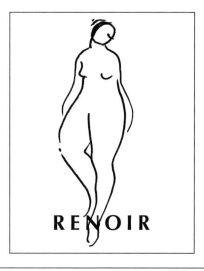

RENOIR

Empire Style Gathered Below Bust

An Ideal Silhouette for the Renoir Shape

This style also suits the Modigliani shape.

■

1. The boat neck widens the shoulder area.

2. Horizontal stripes lead the eye across the shoulders.

3. Short sleeves visually widen the upper torso and balance voluptuous thighs.

4. Gathered below the bust, the skirt gives space for a broader bottom half.

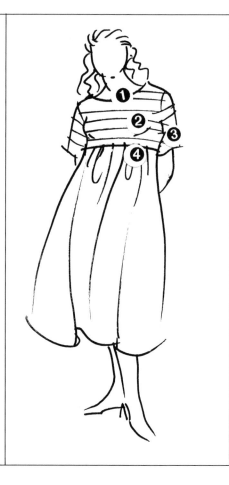

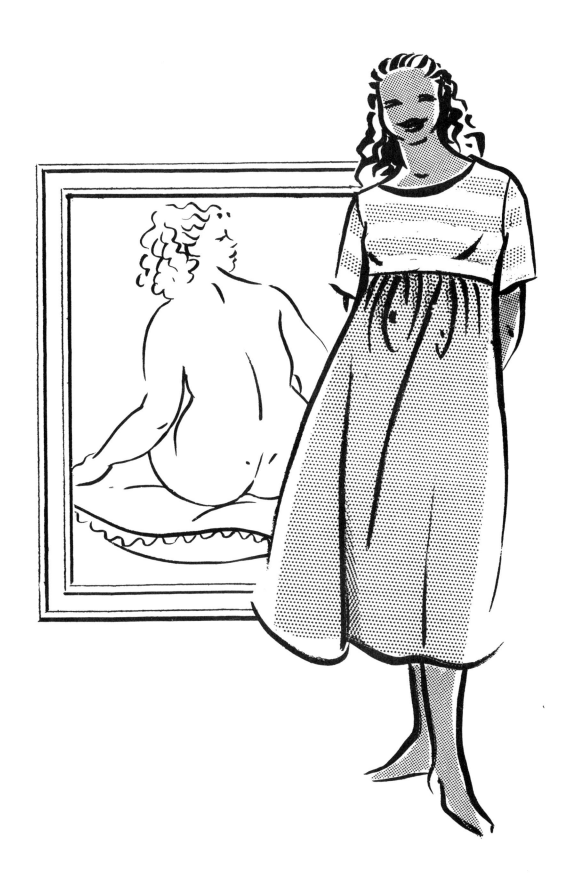

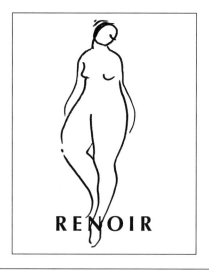

RENOIR

A Long Tent Dress

An Enhancing Silhouette for the Renoir Shape

■

1. Earrings will focus attention close to your face.

2. A wide cowl flatters your feminine décolleté and invites the eye above the waist.

3. The vertical front seam elongates.

4. The unbroken vertical drape gives a stream-lined, slimming silhouette.

5. The A-line gives ease at hips and thighs.

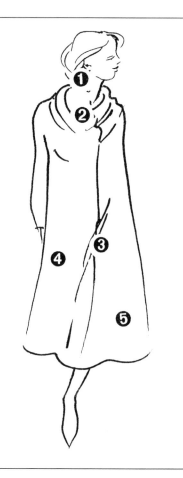

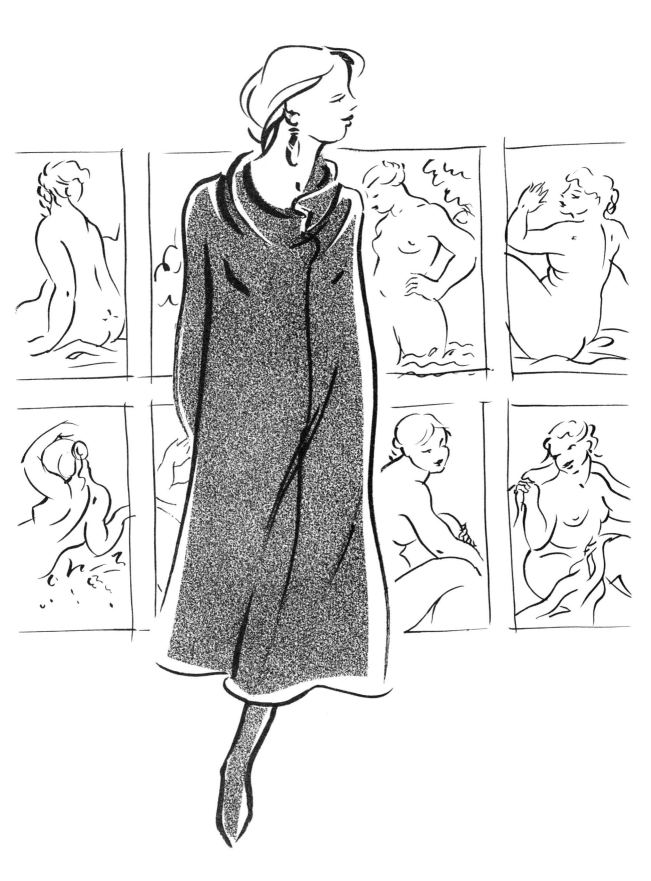

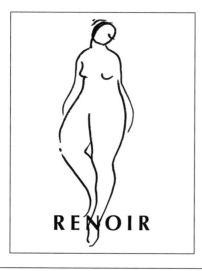

RENOIR

A Semi-Opaque Tunic Over a Black Tubular Knit Dress

A Seductive Combination for the Renoir Shape

This style also suits the Modigliani shape.

∎

1. The black tubular knit under a semi-opaque top layer plays down your curvaceous hips and thighs.

2. The horizontal décolleté of the tubular dress balances your broader bottom half.

3. The top layer in chiffon makes any little bulge invisible.

4. The side-vent of the tunic provides ease at the hip area and visually elongates legs.

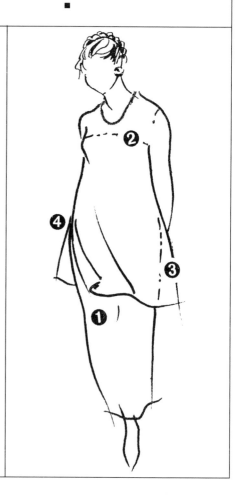

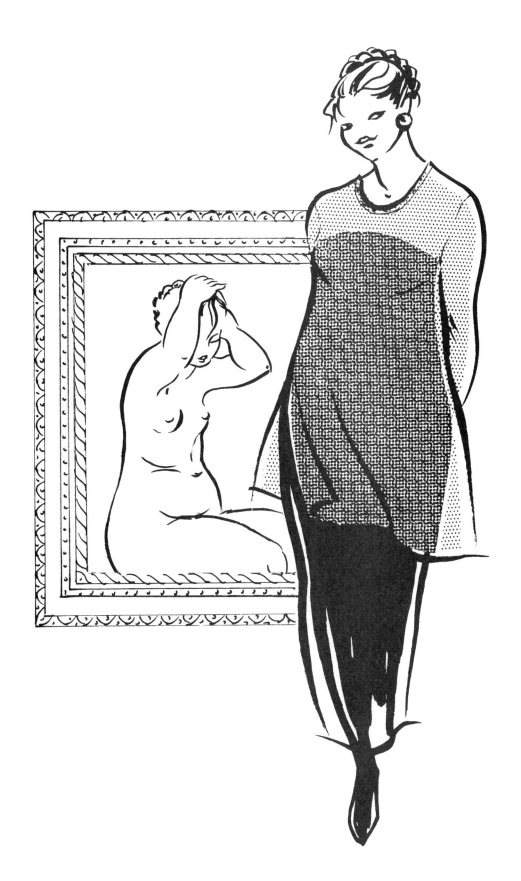

SUMMARY:

Silhouettes that flatter the Renoir shape minimize your figure challenges and show off your assets, and therefore make you look slimmer.

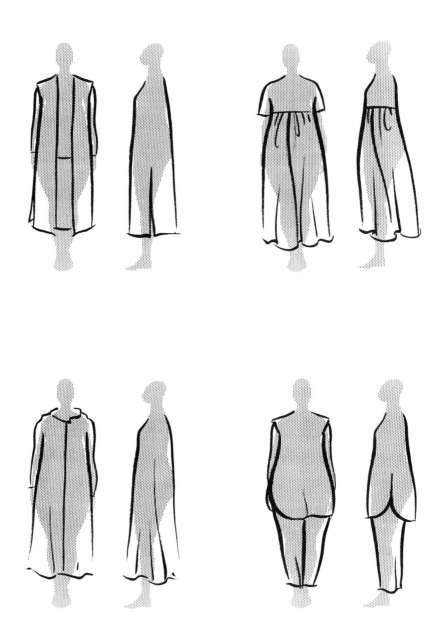

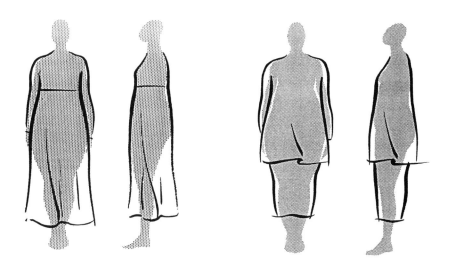

Silhouettes that hide your assets or expose your figure challenges make you look bigger.

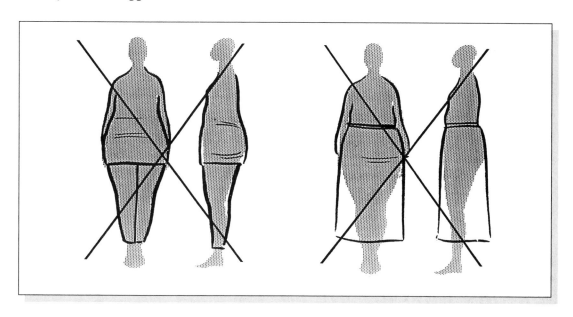

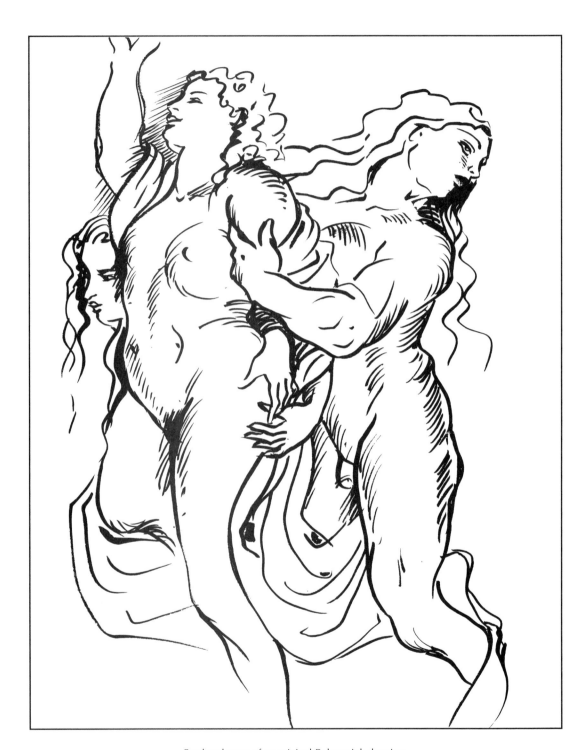

Freehand copy of an original Rubens ink drawing.

rubens

Peter Paul Rubens (1577–1640)

The son of a Protestant lawyer from Antwerp, the young Rubens emigrated to Wesphalia with his family to flee religious persecution. He studied in Wesphalia and in Italy. After the death of his father, he returned to Antwerp, became a Catholic, and opened a very successful studio.

As was common in his time, Rubens was often commissioned to paint for famous people or organizations: Marie de' Medici of France, the Church, the Archduke Albert of Austria, and the Duke of Mantua in Italy, among others.

Rubenesque is a term used liberally to describe women who have an opulent, luscious shape much like the beautiful women of his paintings. Rubens often interprets the human body in a biblical or mythological setting. This is the central theme of his art. His figures exaggerate bodily proportions, especially the upper torso with its ample circumference. In contrast, the lower hips and legs are relatively slender. In this book, I reserve the name of Rubens to illustrate the round figure. The charm and loveliness of his women draw a wide acceptance from his admirers. As a Rubens woman, you are forever mirrored in his work.

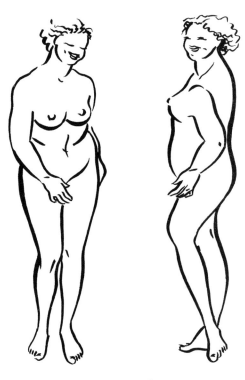

CHARACTERISTICS

1. Ample neck

2. **Generous bust**

3. Wide rib cage

4. Round back

5. **Opulent circumference**

6. Narrow lower hips

7. **Often shapely, slender legs**

Rubens Shape

To Balance and Slenderize Your Silhouette

Visually elongate and slenderize your neck.

■

Downplay your opulent circumference.

■

Lengthen your upper torso.

■

Focus attention to your legs.

Rubens (Round) Shape
General Recommendations

SHAPES AND SILHOUETTES	**Skirts and Pants**	• Straight skirts, provided they are teamed with a long top, in stretch fabrics, knits, or knife pleats will create a narrow silhouette and accentuate your slender lower hips. • Don't hide your assets with bulky or gathered skirts. • Wear any style of pants that create a slim, narrow, straight shape, such as straight, tailored pants, bermudas, stovepipes, or stirrup pants. • Leggings are fine, but only when teamed with a four-fifths-length top. A shorter top would make your upper body look square and heavy in comparison.
	Tops and Dresses	• Jackets should be long and straight, in fabrics that provide a soft, smooth fall but still have body. Dresses have to be loose-fitting and fluid for a streamlined silhouette. • Avoid fitted tops as they will accentuate your large middle. • For more ease at the bust area, dolman sleeves, kimonos, and raglans with comfortable armholes are better than fitted sleeves, but they should never be in a stiff or bulky fabric. • Drapable fabrics will always give you a narrow silhouette, so you don't need to taper your tops toward the hemline. • Wear overblouses or men's shirts unbuttoned.

COLORS AND PRINTS	**Skirts and Pants**	• As your thighs and hips are probably slender, you have the choice in colors and prints for your skirts and pants.
	Tops and Dresses	• For prints, choose medium-sized to large patterns in a low color contrast. Prints that are too small are insignificant for your size. • Avoid bold, loud colors. This does not mean you need to wear only black. Light colors brighten up your face and mood, but wear them in loose-fitting styles and in a soft, drapable fabric only. • If you feel more comfortable in neutral or dark colors, you will need a colorful scarf to brighten up your clothes. • If you wear a jacket and a skirt in the same neutral or deep shade, you can choose a bright color for your blouse. If you wear a dark or neutral color for your blouse and skirt, you can try a bright color for your jacket or cardigan, providing the jacket is unbuttoned. In both options, you will have a continuous color from top to bottom, which lengthens your figure.
FABRICS	**Tops and Dresses**	• Choose soft, supple fabrics for a streamlined look, such as medium-weight knits, soft flannels, crepe, and gabardine. • Avoid stretch fibers, unless worn under a top layer, as they fit too tightly and reveal your ample circumference.

FABRICS (Continued)	**Tops and Dresses** (Continued)	• Stiff fabrics, such as heavy cottons, denim, heavy weaves, raw silk, and taffetas, do not suit you, as they create a silhouette that is too boxy and heavy. Avoid fluffy fabrics, such as fake furs or mohair or any other bulky textures, for the same reason. • Also, beware of synthetic knits that are too fine and have a tendency to cling.
	Skirts and Pants	• Choose either firm fabrics that have body, such as tergal, gabardine, double jersey, burlap, raw silk, linen, brocade, and taffeta, for a loose-fitted, straight line, or fabrics that drape softly around your body and provide a narrow silhouette (for generously cut styles only).
DETAILS	**Tops and Dresses**	• Keep details on your tops to a minimum. • Avoid contrasting colors and shiny or fussy buttons, which would attract attention where you don't want it. • Choose single-breasted rather than double-breasted tops to avoid unnecessary layers. • V necks or elongated, oval necklines will be the best choice for your not-too-slender neck. • For buttoned shirts, leave the first few buttons suggestively undone. Big women have a lovely cleavage. • Avoid collars that are too large, turtlenecks, epaulettes, yokes, breast pockets, horizontal seams, appliqués, and frills.

DETAILS (Continued)	**Tops and Dresses** (Continued)	• Keep collars and lapels narrow and small.
	Skirts and Pants	• To make skirts and pants fit comfortably around your waist, choose elasticized waistbands or, even better, no waistband at all. • Have the darts opened and the waistband cut off to make your skirt sit loosely at or below your natural waistline. Your skirt will no longer pull up in front.
ACCESSORIES	**Handbags**	• Wear the strap of your shoulder bag long enough that your bag will sit at your lower hips. • Avoid backpacks, as they add additional volume to your upper torso. • Belt bags are absolute no-nos. They really would turn your circumference into a focus point.
	Belts	• None!
	Scarves	• Long scarves, draped vertically, in bright colors, will uplift your neutral outfits, bring the attention to your face, and create vertical center-front interest. Just make sure your oblong scarves are long enough to have them hang loosely over your stomach down to your hips.

ACCESSORIES (Continued)	**Scarves** (Continued)	• For extra length, buy two scarves of the same pattern and sew them together. But you could also try two scarves in different colors, such as indigo and burgundy, for instance. This will add additional vertical center-front lines to invite the viewer's eye to pass over your challenges. Anchor the seam with an invisible pin at the center back of your neckline.

TIP: For casual wear, consider shopping in the men's section of your department store. You will find trendy styles in big sizes for a much cheaper price than you would in a specialized shop for big women.

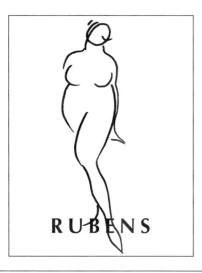

RUBENS

A Long Tunic Paired with a Knife-Pleat Skirt

A Feminine, Elongating Silhouette for the Rubens Shape

This design also flatters the Picasso shape.

■

1. The draped V-neckline elongates your neck.

2. The vertical, top-stiched front seam has a lengthening effect, which makes you appear slimmer.

3. Dropped shoulders give ease to your full bust and back.

4. The loose fit gives room to your voluptuous circumference.

5. Knife pleats in fine knit provide a narrow, streamlined silhouette and flatter your legs because of the skirt's flippy movement.

TIP: *Wear a camisole under your top, but let it float **over** your waistband instead of tucking it in. This way, your top won't cling to your skirt and will drape better.*

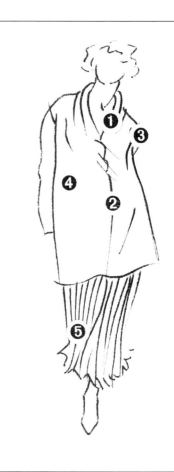

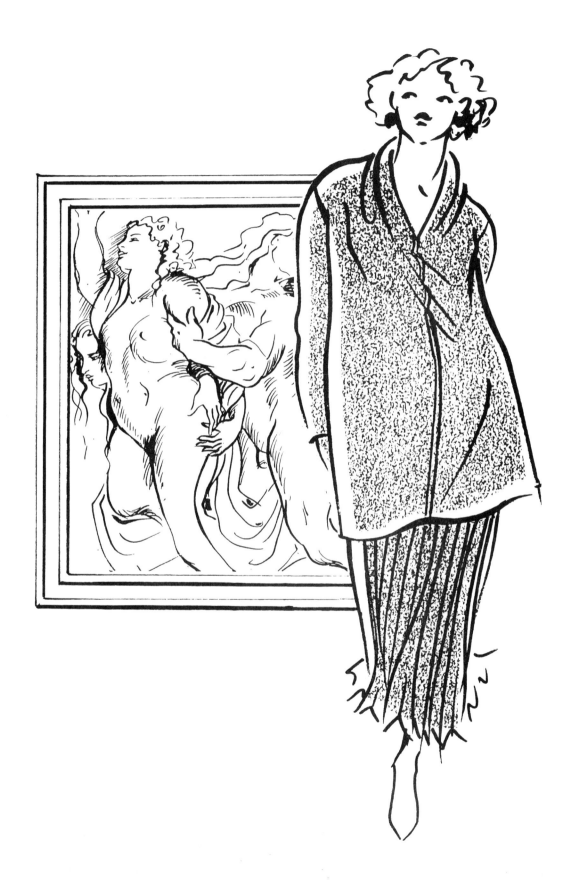

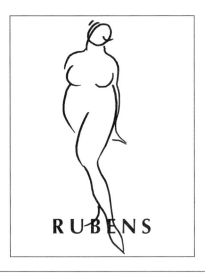

RUBENS

Safari Jacket Teamed with a Skirt or Straight, Narrow Pants

A Classic Silhouette for the Rubens Shape

Can also be worn by the Picasso and Gauguin shapes.

■

1. The notch collar provides an open neckline.

2. The generous, loose fit of this jacket gives enough room to your upper torso.

3. With your narrow lower hips, you can afford patch pockets.

NOTE: *Always wear your contrasting-colored jacket unbuttoned over a single-colored outfit. This will create a long, monochromatic center-front panel to lengthen your silhouette and avoid an unattractive horizontal division.*

This jacket also mixes well with straight, narrow pants.

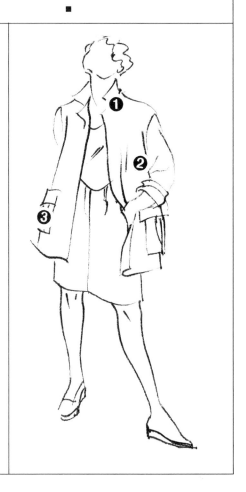

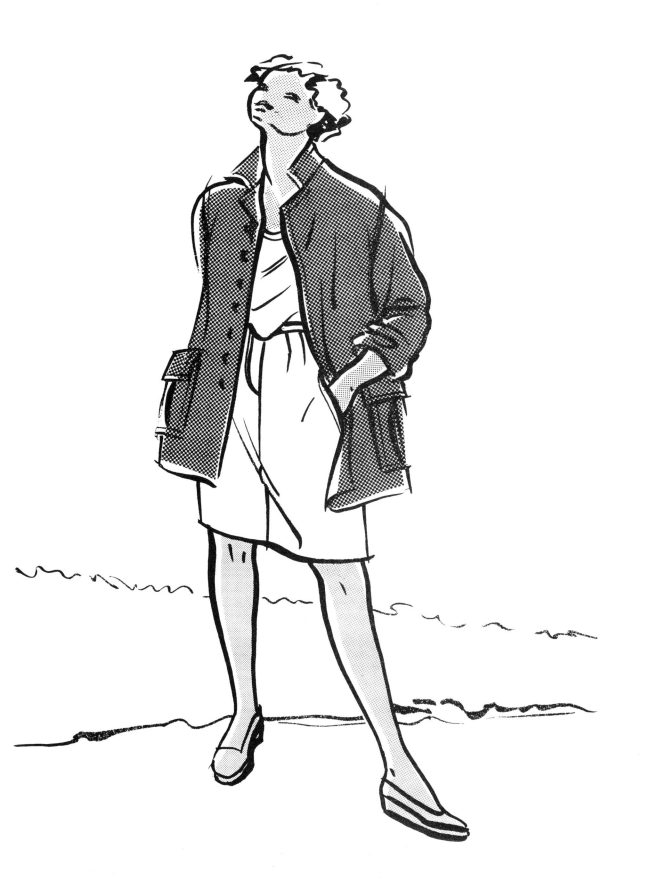

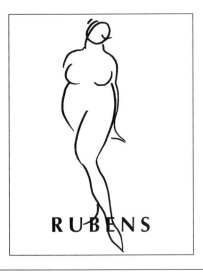

RUBENS

Three-Quarter-Length Jacket Teamed with a Long, Narrow Skirt

A Flattering Silhouette for the Rubens Shape

This also suits the Picasso and Gauguin shapes.

■

1. The V neck provides a slimming, open neck-line.

2. An oblong loose-hanging scarf creates vertical, center-front interest and visually lengthens the upper torso.

3. The large-scaled motif of the skirt invites the eye to your slender bottom half.

4. The scarf matched to your skirt has a lengthening effect.

NOTE: This jacket also looks great with a shorter skirt or with long, narrow pants.

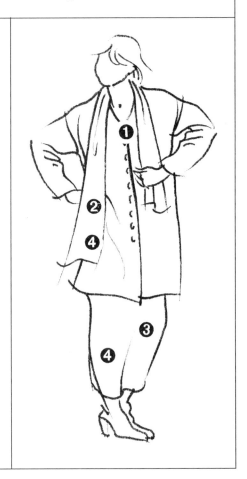

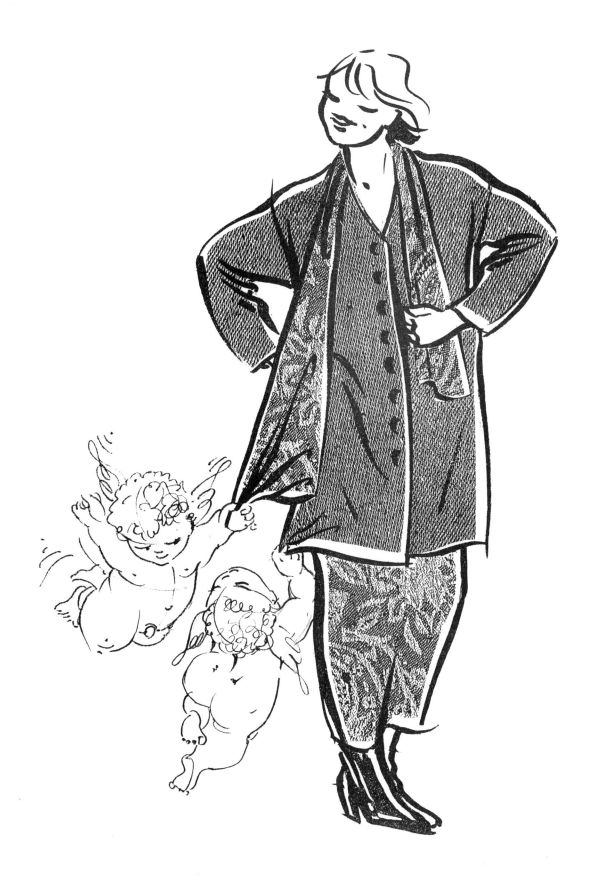

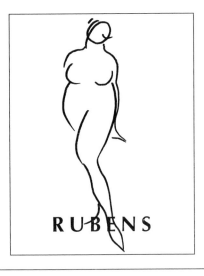

RUBENS

A Fine-Knit Tunic Over a Layered, Sheer Skirt

A Relaxed Silhouette with a Romantic Note for the Rubens Shape

A style that also suits the Gauguin shape.

■

1. The straight, loosely fitted tunic in a fine knit floats over your skirt and provides a streamlined look.

2. The layered, sheer skirt in chiffon keeps the silhouette narrow. The fabric moves as you move and makes you look and feel so light... like you are almost dancing.

NOTE: *For a better drape, always wear a camisole beneath a fine knit. The camisole should be three to four inches shorter than your tunic so you can let it fall over your skirt instead of tucking it into your waistband.*

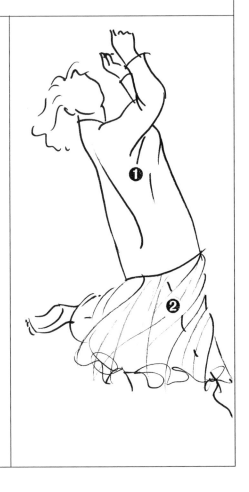

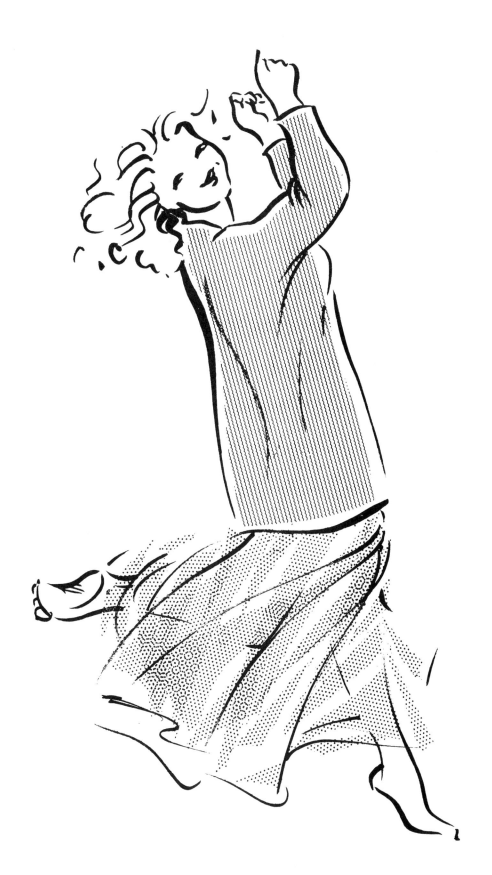

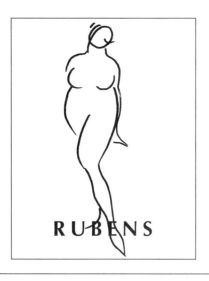

RUBENS

A Wedge Dress

A Casual, Streamlined Silhouette for the Rubens Shape

This style also suits the Picasso shape.

∎

1. A kimono, low-cut under the arm, gives fullness to your bustline.

2. A large-scale motif looks great on big women, providing the color contrast between the motif and background is subdued.

3. Closely spaced buttons create a desired vertical line.

4. Side vents reveal well-shaped legs.

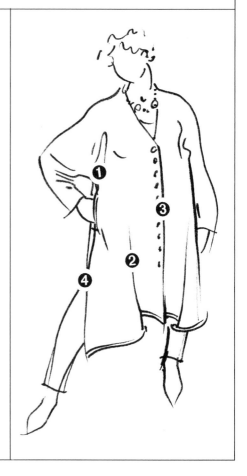

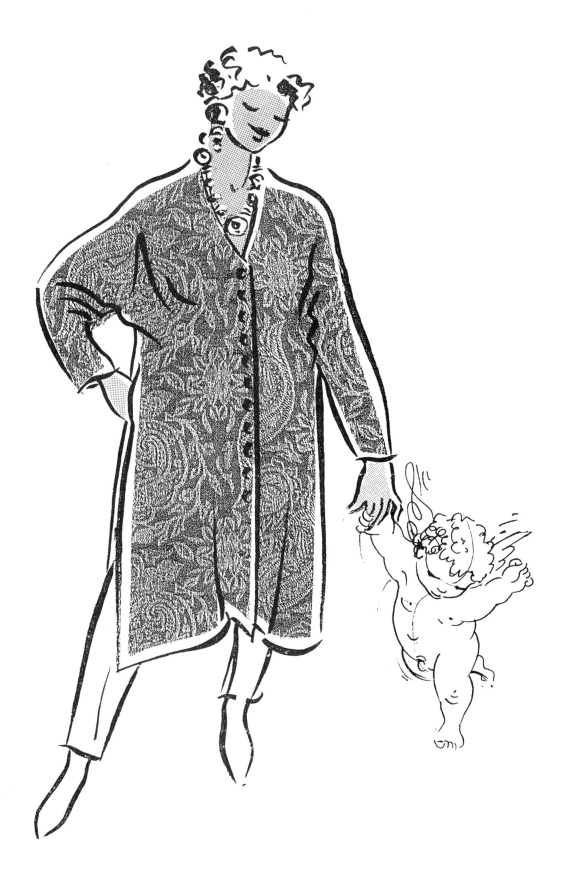

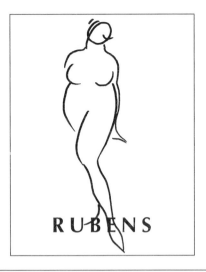

RUBENS

A Black Dress As a Slimming Base for a Sheer, Chiffon Jacket

This style also enhances the Picasso shape.

■

1. Black, the most receding color, plays down your Baroque curves.

2. The Lycra-rayon blend of the dress offers a sleek fit that gives.

3. The long side vent adds a sexy edge and draws attention to well-shaped legs.

4. A sheer top layer over a deeply colored base flatters most bodies. The floppy movement and the transparency of the fabric lends a feather-light dimension to your silhouette ... and makes you feel you are flying.

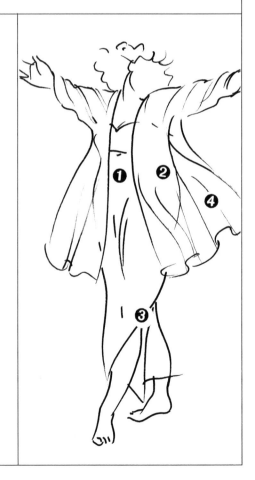

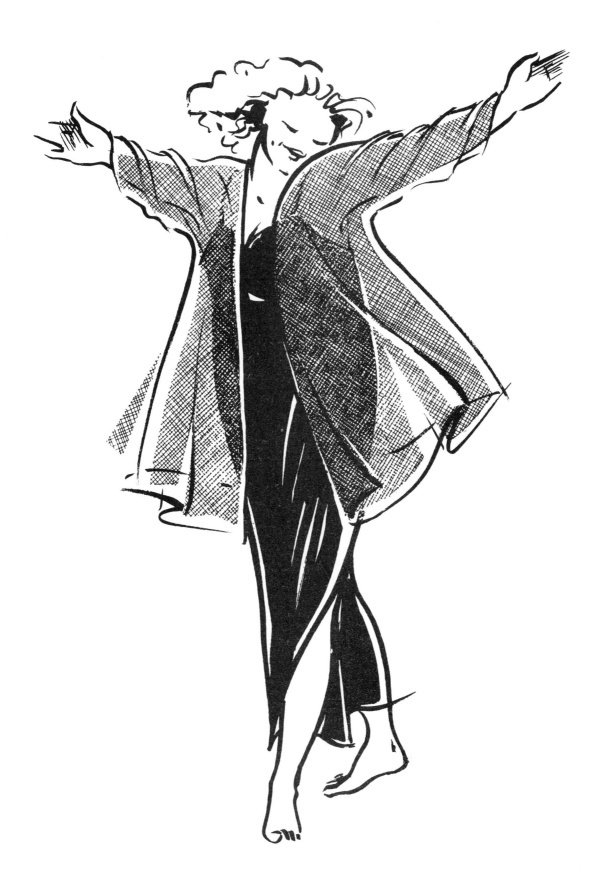

SUMMARY:

Silhouettes that flatter the Rubens shape minimize your figure challenges, show off your assets, and therefore make you look slimmer.

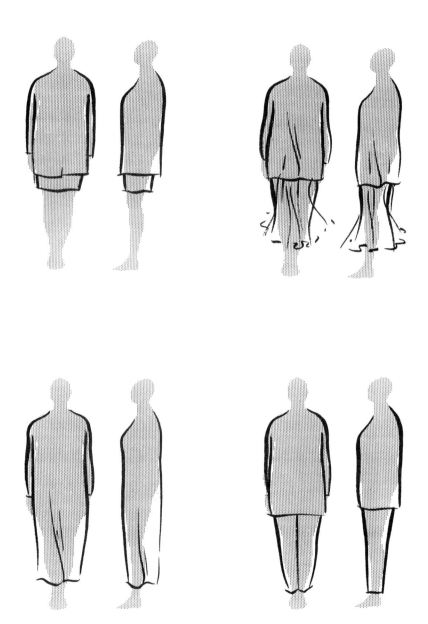

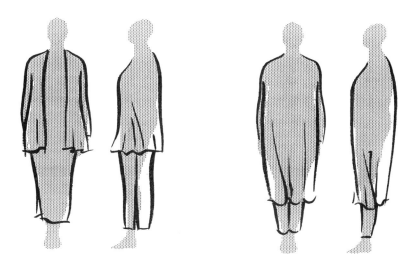

Silhouettes that hide your assets or expose your figure challenges make you look bigger.

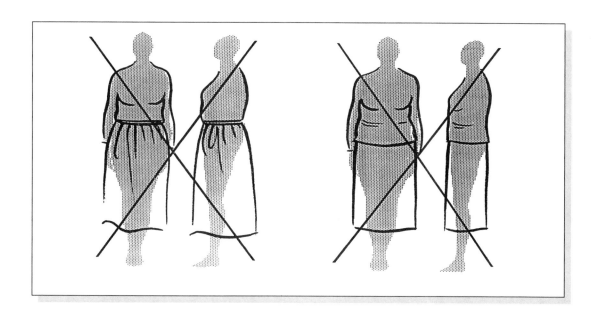

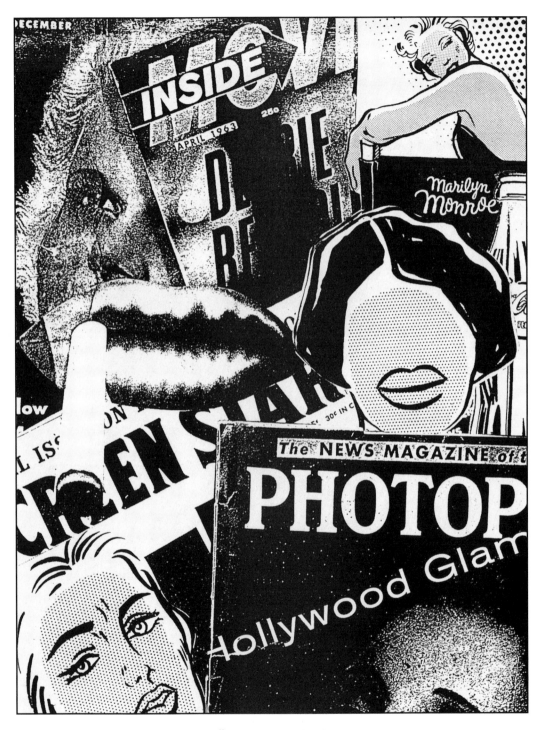

Collage representing Pop Art.

CHAPTER FIVE

pop art

Pop Art (1950 . . .)

Fascination for pop (for *populist*) art originated in England in the mid-fifties at the Institute of Contemporary Art. Although it began in England, pop art was actually related to new, truly American cultural phenomena: comic strips, canned foods, soft drinks, advertising, and wide-screen Hollywood movies. It is the first art movement to be seen by both international admirers and critics as really representing the American culture of modern times.

Works of pop artists, such as Andy Warhol, Roy Lichtenstein, Tom Wesselman, and Robert Rauschenberg, conjure up the classic period of Hollywood stars like Marilyn Monroe, the curvaceous women with generous hips and breasts and a highly defined waist. Therefore, I have renamed the hourglass shape the pop art shape, after the entire movement. If this is you, you are forever idealized in pop art and the Hollywood films of the fifties.

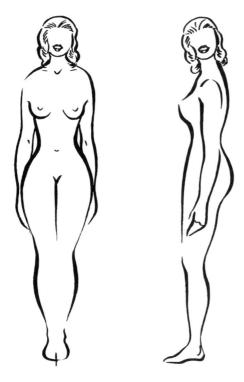

CHARACTERISTICS

1. Delicate bone structure

2. **Pronounced bust**

3. **Defined waist**

4. **Curved hips**

5. Sometimes, protruding buttocks

6. Shapely legs

Pop Art Shape

To Enhance and Balance Your Silhouette

Draw attention to your waist.

∎

Play up your curves with soft, drapable fabrics.

∎

Don't disguise your delicate bone structure with oversized or loose-fitting styles.

Pop Art (Hourglass) Shape
General Recommendations

SHAPES AND SILHOUETTES	Skirts and Pants	<ul><li>With that dream figure of yours, show off your waist; choose high waistbands for your pants and skirts and contrasting colored belts. But don't cinch your waist if your curves are too Baroque.</li><li>Your skirts can be straight, in stretch fibers, if your behind is not too protruding; otherwise, wear skirts with an unbuttoned jacket or opt for styles slightly eased at the waist.</li><li>Use soft, fluid fabrics that hug your curves. These are ideal for pants, too.</li><li>A sarong or wrap skirt will look great on you.</li><li>Hip huggers teamed with a cropped top will expose your beautiful waist.</li><li>Tiered skirt? Yes, but only if you are medium or tall in height and if your buttocks are not protruding. Too much volume at the bottom would make you look shorter.</li><li>A pronounced waist will accentuate your curves, so, if your bust is on the generous side, overblouse your tops slightly.</li><li>You look great in a wrap dress, which will drape around your body and accentuate your feminine shape.</li><li>Semifitted tunics or dresses in medium-weight knits or soft, drapable fabrics are also ideal and will hint at your curves without overaccentuating your bust and hips. If you are short in height, this would be your best choice.</li></ul>

SHAPES AND SILHOUETTES (Continued)	Tops and Dresses	• *Keep in mind that semifitted styles that are slightly waisted are more slimming and lengthening and show off a curved figure to better advantage than tightly fitted garments.* • Avoid oversized, bulky, or stiff clothes that will disguise your thin waist and fine bone structure and will make you look bigger than you actually are.
COLORS AND PRINTS	Tops and Bottoms	• You look best when you wear the same color from head to toe. This will play up your balanced figure. • If you are on the taller side and if your curves are not too impressive, you can wear a contrasting colored belt to focus attention on your waistline. • For prints, select medium- to small-scaled, feminine prints. • Beware of stripes or linear geometric designs. They won't complement your rounded body shape.
FABRICS	Skirts and Pants	• For fitted styles, use stretch fibers such as Lycra, spandex, or blends. They are flexible, light, and mold over curves. Wear them teamed with an open jacket if your curves are too generous. • For semifitted or draped styles, opt for soft, drapable fabrics such as knits, jerseys, fluid microfibers, washed silk, viscose, loose weaves, chiffons, wool crepes, challis, fluid satin, velvets, and rayon.

FABRICS (Continued)	**Tops and Dresses**	• Here again, use fabrics that will drape well around your body. • Avoid stiff, crisp, tight weaves, especially for fitted styles, as they will just make you look bigger.
DETAILS	**Skirts and Pants**	• A tight waistband will show off your tiny waist to advantage but accentuate your bust and butt. • As you want to focus attention to your middle, leave your skirts and pants as plain as possible.
	Tops and Dresses	• Keep your collars and neckline soft. • Shawl collars, cowl necks, turtlenecks, tuxedos, crossovers, round necklines, sweetheart openings, keyholes, off-shoulder styles, gathered necklines, and strapless dresses all suit your body shape and, if you are in a daring mood, a deep décolleté shows off your lovely cleavage (for evening or beachwear only).
ACCESSORIES	**Shoes**	• With your delicate bone structure, you probably have fine ankles, so opt for feminine, delicate styles such as pumps, slingbacks, slides, delicate ankle straps, wedges, ballerinas, and mules. • For boots, choose laced, fitted ones. • Steer clear of chunky shoes with heavy soles. • Go for medium to high heels (2"–4" or 5–10 cm)

ACCESSORIES (Continued)	**Shoes** (Continued)	depending on your outfit. Spikes at work, however, are out of place. • For flat heels, select the delicate ballerina type.
	Handbags	• Soft, medium-sized bags will look best on you. • Shoulder bags should not be too sporty. • For work, opt for a medium-sized, soft, unstructured tote. • For the evening, a clutch bag or a small string bag will be fine. • Keep the colors of your bag neutral; save any eye-catching color as a focal point for your waist.
	Belts	• Yes, of course! Belt your tiny waist. • Play with contrasting colors to focus attention to your waist. • With your shapely middle, you can wear any height of belt, unless your upper torso is really short. • A sash, an obi, or any waist wrap made out of a colorful scarf will flatter your figure. • If your curves are too obvious, add an open top layer.

ACCESSORIES (Continued)	**Scarves**	• Choose soft, fluid, or transparent scarves in plain colors that flatter your skin tone or with soft, delicate, flower prints, polka dots, or soft abstracts.
	Jewelry	• Forget about brooches, unless you put them at your waist. • You probably look best in precious luxury jewelry, such as antique jewelry, filigree, pearls, precious or semiprecious stones. • Avoid pendants if your bust is too generous. Instead, select a delicate necklace that falls just below the base of your neck.

TIP: *Why not scatter a few studs or pins on your belt or waistband. It will make your waist the focal point of your figure.*

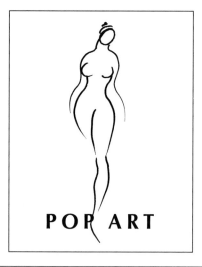

POP ART

A Simple T-Dress

**Hints at Your Waist Without Emphasizing
Your Curves**

■

1. The simple, semifitted, little black dress in a
   nonclinging, fine knit gives you an unbroken,
   streamlined silhouette.

2. The deep, round neckline suits your curved
   body shape.

3. No details are necessary when only the
   essential is needed to play up your balanced
   figure.

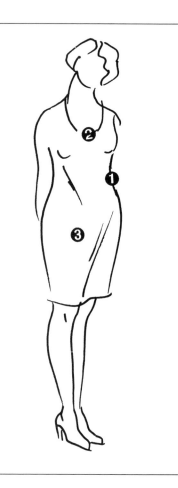

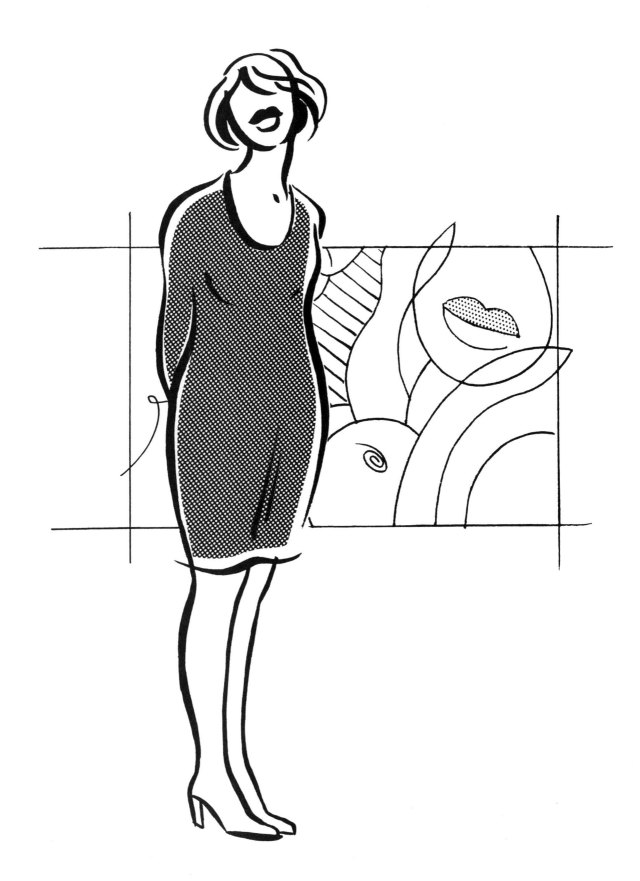

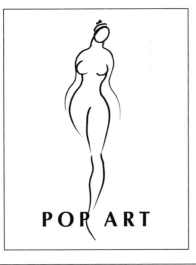

P O P A R T

This Feminine Suit

Provides a Shapely Lined Silhouette for the Pop Art Figure

This style also suits the Modigliani shape.

■

1. The soft shawl collar enhances your décolleté.

2. A hint of a lace camisole for a touch of sex appeal.

3. Semifitted, so as not to hide your delicate bone structure and fine waist.

4. A skirt that falls above the knee teamed with a jacket that ends just below the buttocks provides a balanced proportion for the pop art shape.

NOTE: *This jacket can also be paired with a long, fluid, narrow skirt or pants.*

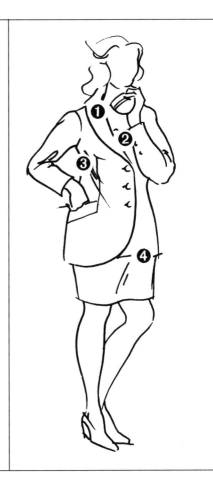

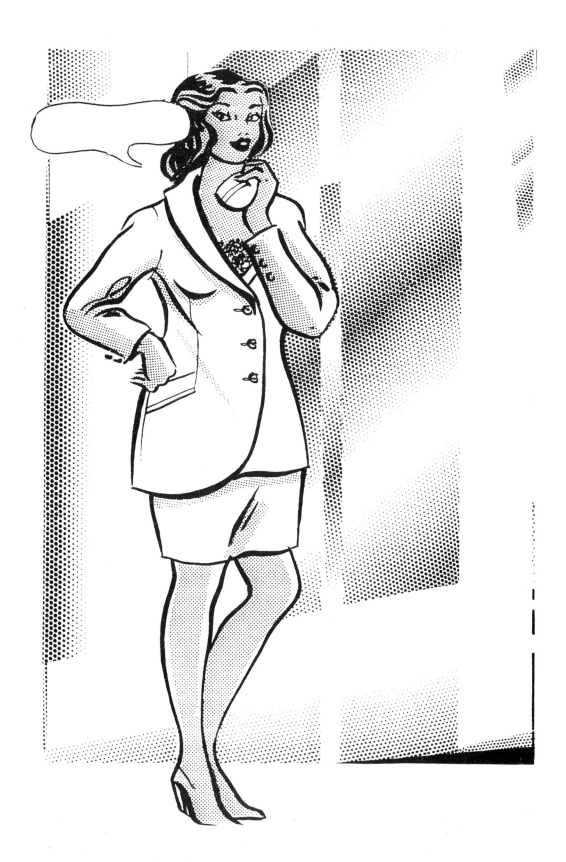

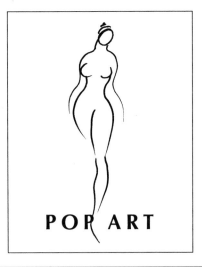

POP ART

The Belted Pullover Dress

A Relaxed but Curve-Conscious Silhouette for the Pop Art Figure (If Medium to Tall in Height)

■

1. Raglan sleeves give room for a full bust.

2. Overblouse to play down a generous bust-line.

3. Contrasting-colored belt to accentuate and highlight your delicate waist.

4. The belted straight dress gives ease at hip area.

NOTE: For a loose or baggy style, always wear a belt so as not to hide your best feature, your waist. Wear it tight or, if your curves are too pro-nounced, sling it loosely around the waist.

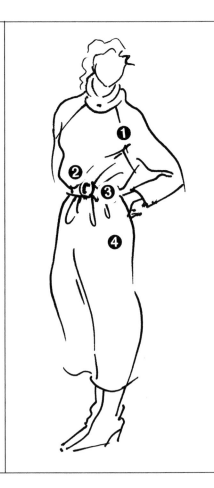

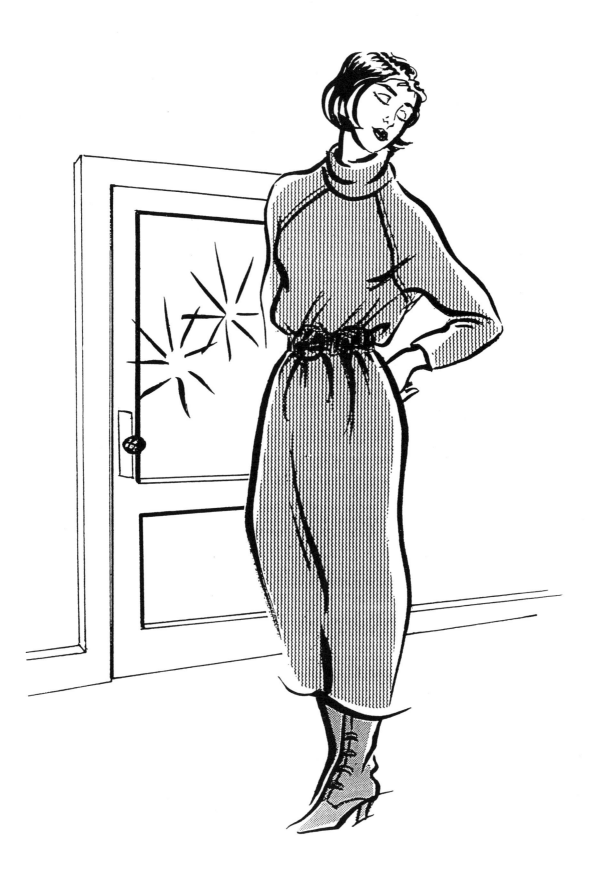

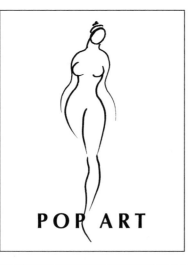

POP ART

A Simple Knotted Shirt
Teamed with Hip Huggers

**A Silhouette That Enhances the Pop Art Figure
(Avoid If Long-Waisted)**

■

1. The suggestively undone buttons give a sexy note to a masculine shirt.

2. Knotted at waist level to invite the eye to your best feature, your waist, and to deemphasize your full bust.

3. Hip huggers reveal a generous butt less than does a cinched waist.

NOTE: *Jeans in a cotton-Lycra blend stretch easily over your curves for a tight fit, yet expand when necessary.*

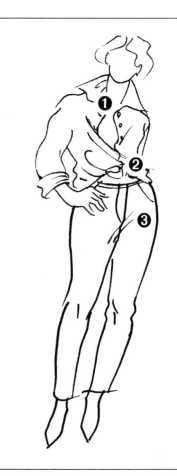

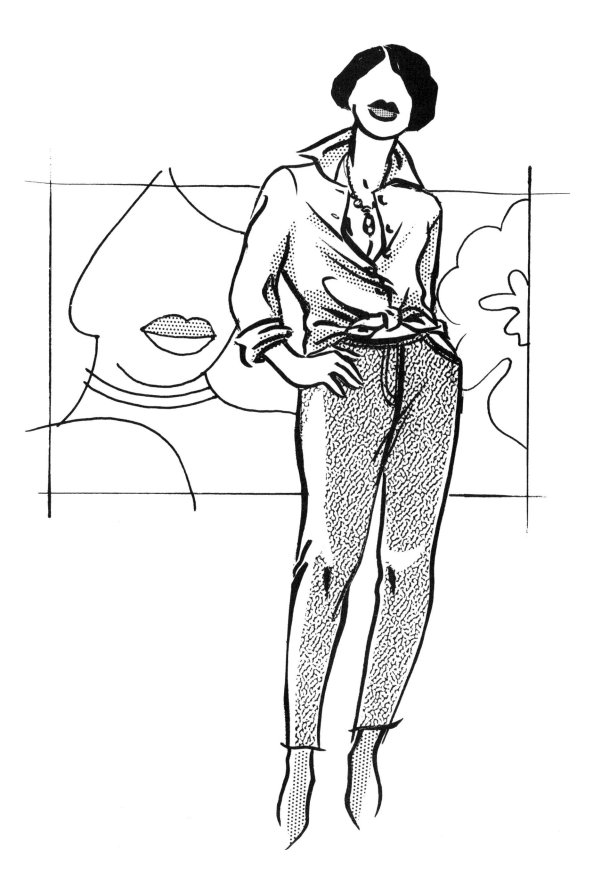

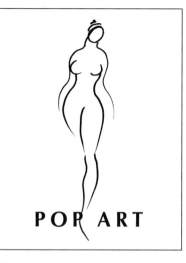

POP ART

The Body-Hugging
Wrap Dress

A Feminine Silhouette for the Pop Art Figure

*This style also suits the
Modigliani shape.*

■

1. A deep, crossover V neck slenderizes the bustline.

2. The asymmetrical drape gives room for bust and hips.

3. Tied at waist level to keep the wrap dress in place and turn your waist into a focal point.

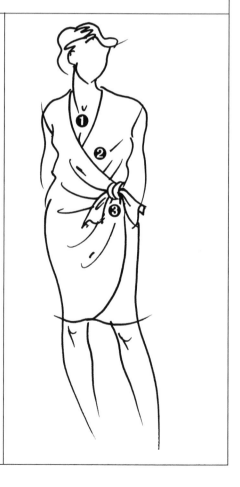

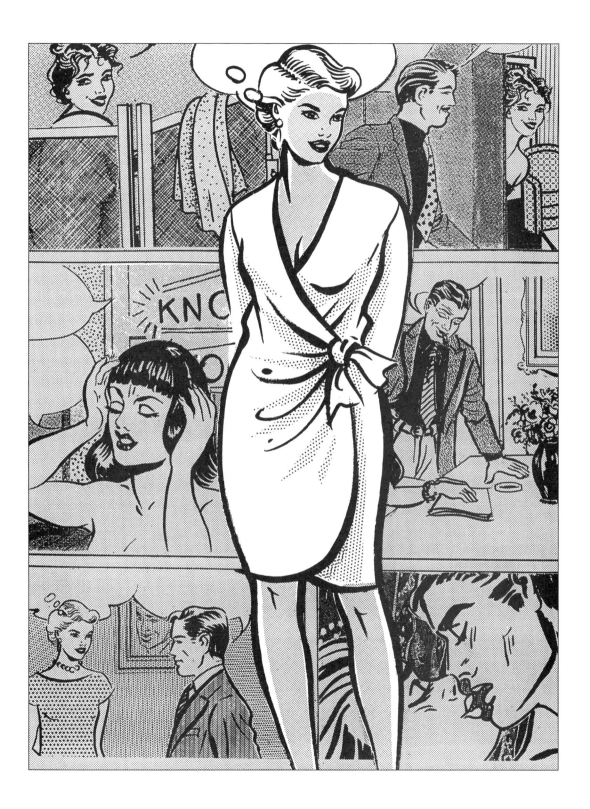

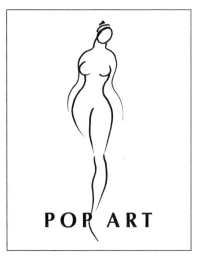

POP ART

A Strong, Sexy Statement with the Classic, Body-Caressing Satin Halter-Neck Dress

The Most Feminine Pop Art Silhouette for a Night on the Town

1. The draped halter neckline gives ease to a full bust.

2. Cut on the bias for a perfect drape.

3. The vertical drape of the halter neckline and the center-front seam provide an elongating, unbroken, streamlined silhouette.

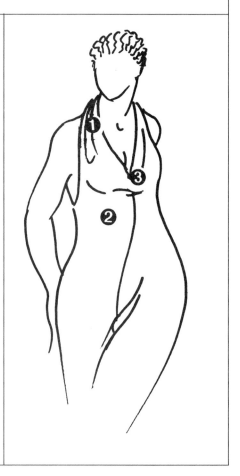

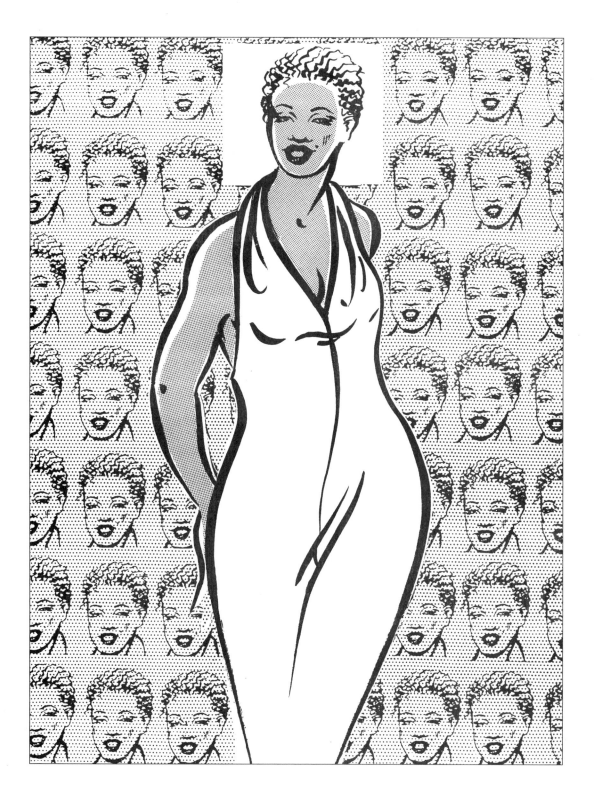

SUMMARY:

Silhouettes that flatter the pop art shape minimize your figure challenges, show off your assets, and therefore make you look slimmer.

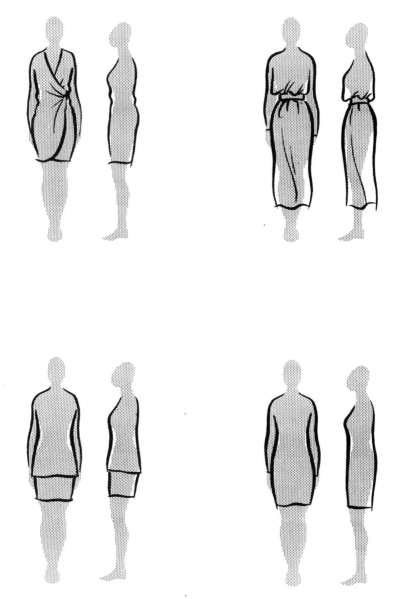

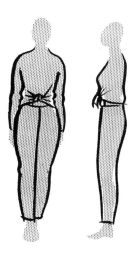 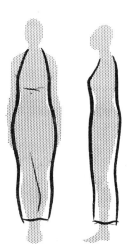

Silhouettes that hide your assets or expose your figure challenges make you look bigger.

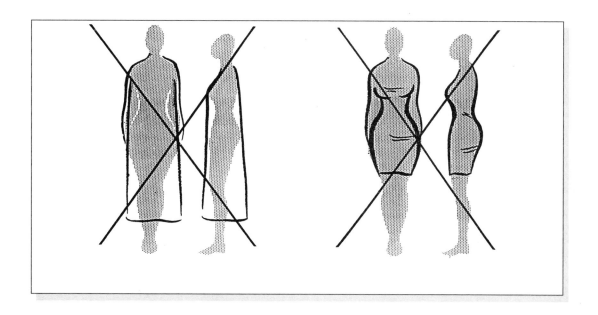

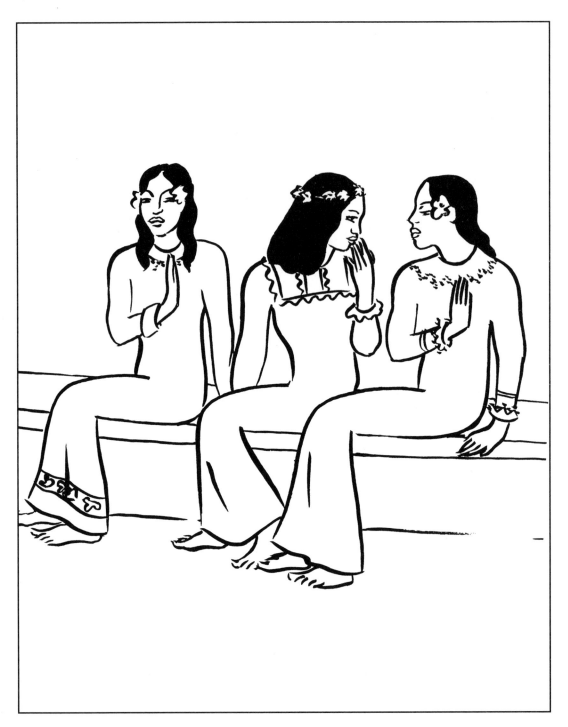

Line drawing inspired by Gauguin's painting *We Shall Not Go to Market Today*.

gauguin

Paul Gauguin (1848–1903)

Born in Paris, Gauguin was the son of a Peruvian-Creole mother and a French journalist. When the future Napoléon III came to power in 1849, Gauguin's republican father went into exile to Peru with his family. Gauguin returned to France as a young man, where he spent six years as a sailor, worked in the stock exchange in Paris until the crash of 1882, and painted part time.

At thirty-four, he became a full-time painter in Paris, in Britanny, in Arles with his friend van Gogh, and finally in the South Seas, where he died at age fifty-four.

Gauguin's stylized paintings capture the harmony of humankind and nature. In his work, he reconciles the physical grace of the androgynous and the exotic femininity of the Tahitian women. I gave his name to the inverted triangle shape because he celebrates women with wide shoulders and narrow hips; yet another example of beauty. You can see them walking straight and proud along the beaches of Tahiti. If you are a Gauguin shape, then carry yourself with the same sensual dignity as the beautiful Tahitians.

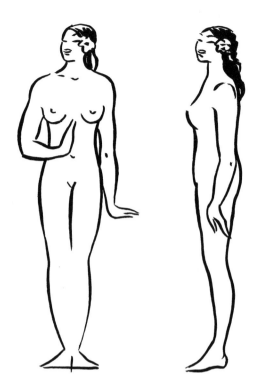

Gauguin Shape

CHARACTERISTICS

1. *Broad shoulders*

2. Medium to full bust

3. Average waist

4. *Narrow hips*

5. Shapely, long legs

To Enhance and Balance Your Silhouette

Focus attention on your slender hips.

▪

Emphasize your long, shapely legs.

▪

Minimize your shoulder area.

▪

Downplay your upper torso.

Gauguin (Inverted Triangle) Shape
General Recommendations

SHAPES AND SILHOUETTES	**Skirts**	▪ For your shape, you can wear any skirt you choose, except ones that are too full (gathered at the waist or with open pleats), as this would disguise your slender bottom half. ▪ Wear straight flared, gored, circular, A-line, trumped, or wrapped skirts. This will create silhouettes that show off your fine hips. Tiered skirts are fine if the gathering starts at hip level.
	Pants	▪ You look great in trousers! From narrow to wide, from fluid to crisp, from short to long, you can't go wrong. Hip huggers, jeans, stovepipes, culottes, shorts, cuffed pants, bell-bottoms, and palazzo pants all suit your figure. ▪ Of course, wear leggings, if teamed with the right top. Leggings should always be coordinated with fluid, long tops in proportion to your narrow hips. ▪ The question of proportion and harmony should be a priority.
	Tops and Dresses	▪ Beware of tightly-fitted bodices. You don't want to emphasize your upper torso. ▪ Loose, unstructured, fluid tops will best feminize your sporty figure. ▪ You don't need any shoulder pads.

SHAPES AND SILHOUETTES (Continued)	**Tops and Dresses** (Continued)	• If you wish to emphasize your athletic figure with a sporty jacket or suit, play with masculine/feminine contrasts. For instance, match the jacket with a feminine blouse in soft, fluid satin or another drapable fabric for a sophisticated Armani look. • Deep armholes (raglan, kimono, and dropped sleeves) will give you additional ease at the bust area and deemphasize your square shoulders, providing the fabric is soft and drapable for a streamlined silhouette. • The best type of dresses for you are shirtdresses with a hip sash or hip belt, coat dresses, dropped waists, pullover dresses, tunics, a wedge, or a sheath dress.
COLORS AND PRINTS	**Tops and Bottoms**	• Wear deep or neutral colors above the waist to make your upper torso look smaller. These can be brightened up with colorful accessories. • Keep bright, bold colors or big prints for the bottom in order to draw attention to your slender hips and legs.
FABRICS	**Tops and Dresses**	• For your tops, choose drapable, medium-weight fabrics, such as jersey, knits, crepe, soft flannel, and loose weaves for an unstructured, feminine look. A loosely fitted, straight-line style, such as a jacket, demands a firmer, tighter weave, such as tergal, linen, serge, herringbone, light tweed, double knit, gabardine, etc.

FABRICS (Continued)	**Skirts and Pants**	• Wear any type of fabric, depending upon the silhouette you desire. • Wear soft, fluid fabrics for flared, gored, circular, or wrapped skirts and softly gathered or palazzo pants. • For a more structured fit, such as hip huggers, jeans, stovepipes, culottes, shorts, cuffed pants, and straight skirts, choose firm textures such as gabardine, linen, cotton, natural silk, tergal, mixed fibers, Lycra, or denim.
DETAILS	**Tops & Dresses**	• Avoid double-breasted tops, breast pockets, horizontal seams, trimmings, and piping. These all draw attention to your bust. • For a slimming illusion, wear V necks, single-breasted tops, small lapels, narrow, small collars, oblong scarves, necklaces, and pendants. • Use vertical seams, trimmings, and piped edges, if in style, to make the eye move up and down. This will help to slenderize your upper torso. • Leave the top as plain as possible and keep details for below the waist. • Don't wear boat necks, large lapels, or gathered sleeves or yokes, as these will create the illusion that your shoulders are wider than they are.
	Skirts and Pants	• Wear belts, yokes, gatherings, and patch pockets at the hip area.

DETAILS (Continued)	Skirts and Pants (Continued)	▪ Horizontal trimmings and boarder prints bring the eye down to your slender legs.
ACCESSORIES	Shoes	▪ With your long, well-shaped legs, you can play with different styles and designs, depending upon the current trend. ▪ From high to flat and heavy to narrow heels, you have the choice. ▪ Avoid spikes, straps that are too thin, small buckles, bows, and ties; in short, any dainty, small details. They don't suit your athletic look. ▪ You look stunning in any type of boots, high or low, depending on the length of your skirt.
	Handbags	▪ You could wear a shoulder bag, a tote, a backpack, or belt bag (at hip level). Bags that are too small, with fancy details, look too cute with your build. ▪ Keep bags in neutral colors so you can wear them with everything. ▪ Bags do not have to match your shoes, but they should match the look of your outfit.
	Belts	▪ Keep belts neutral or of the same color as your garment, so as not to draw attention to your not-too-defined waist. ▪ Never wear light-colored belts, as this would make your middle appear wider.

ACCESSORIES (Continued)	**Belts** (Continued)	• Buckles should be simple. • Wear your belts loosely around your waist, and have your top bloused over, or sling one belt or multiple belts around hipbone level, for a more casual look. This will focus attention on your assets, your hips. A hip sash will yield similar results.
	Scarves	• Long scarves worn vertically create vertical lines for an elongating, streamlined look. • A man's tie (if in fashion) will suit your style, but tie it loosely and match it with one or two strings of pearls. • Beware of flower prints that are too small. Play around with bright colors to brighten your neutral tops. • Plaids, stripes, geometrics, abstract prints, and ethnic prints will suit your figure type best.
	Jewelry	• Fantasy jewelry in geometric designs, ethnic jewelry if in fashion, and simple metal, wood, or plastic jewelry will suit your style better than jewelry that is too tiny and delicate. • Wear necklaces long and pendants just above your waist, never at bust level. You don't need a focus point in that area.

TIP: *Wear your brooches, pendants, and ear clips on your hips. Yes, on your hips! This is an original way to keep your hip sash or wrap skirt in place and to focus attention on your slender bottom half.*

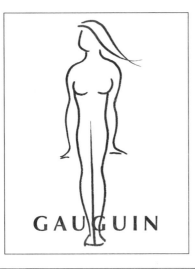

GAUGUIN

Shirtdress with a Loosely Draped Sash Below the Waistline

A Flattering Silhouette for the Gauguin Shape

This silhouette also suits the Pop Art figure.

■

1. Small collar lapels lengthen the neckline.

2. High, set-in sleeves visually narrow wide shoulders.

3. Single front opening slenderizes.

4. Sash below natural waistline elongates upper torso and disguises full bust.

5. The same colored sash does not break the dress horizontally.

6. Patch pockets balance wide shoulders.

7. Hemline above knee to show off shapely legs.

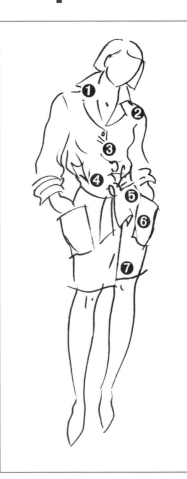

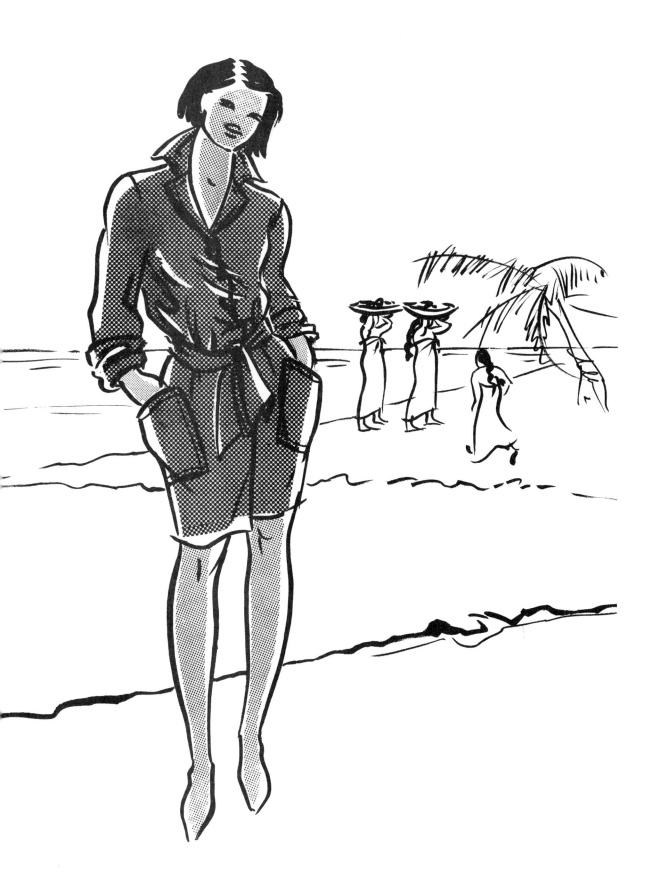

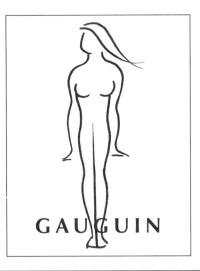

GAUGUIN

An Overbloused, Tucked-In Top Matched with a Flared Skirt

An Excellent Choice for the Gauguin Shape

■

1. The V neck provides an open neckline.

2. Kimono sleeves soften straight or angular shoulders and give ease at the bust area.

3. A loosely fitted, overbloused, fine-knit tunic creates the illusion of a longer waist.

4. A skirt that sits below the waist is a perfect choice for an undefined waist.

5. A low-slung chain belt dresses up any skirt and attracts attention to your hips.

6. The skirt is fitted at hip level to invite the eye to your assets.

7. The flared skirt balances wide shoulders (best worn with a medium to high heel).

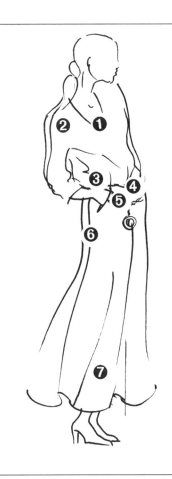

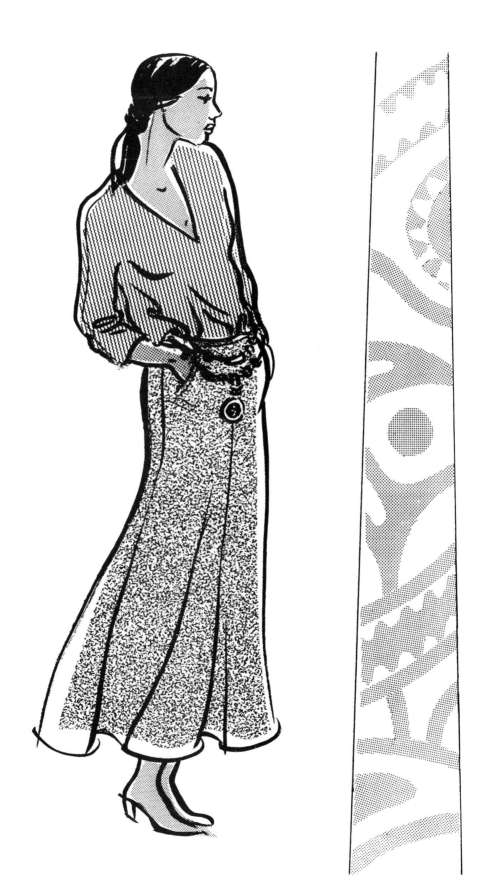

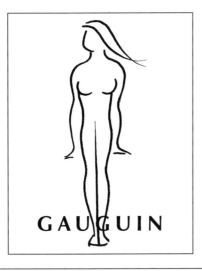

GAUGUIN

A Straight, Three-Quarters-Length Jacket Paired with a Miniskirt

A Good Proportion for the Gauguin Shape

This silhouette also suits the Picasso shape.

■

1. Narrow, set-in sleeves downplay the shoulder area.

2. The notch-collar creates an elongated neckline.

3. A long, oblong scarf creates center-front vertical lines and distracts attention from shoulder area.

4. Stripes at both ends of the scarf bring the eye to your slender bottom half.

5. The long, straight jacket lengthens your upper torso, even more so if paired with a short skirt.

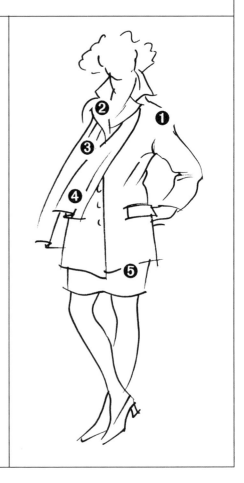

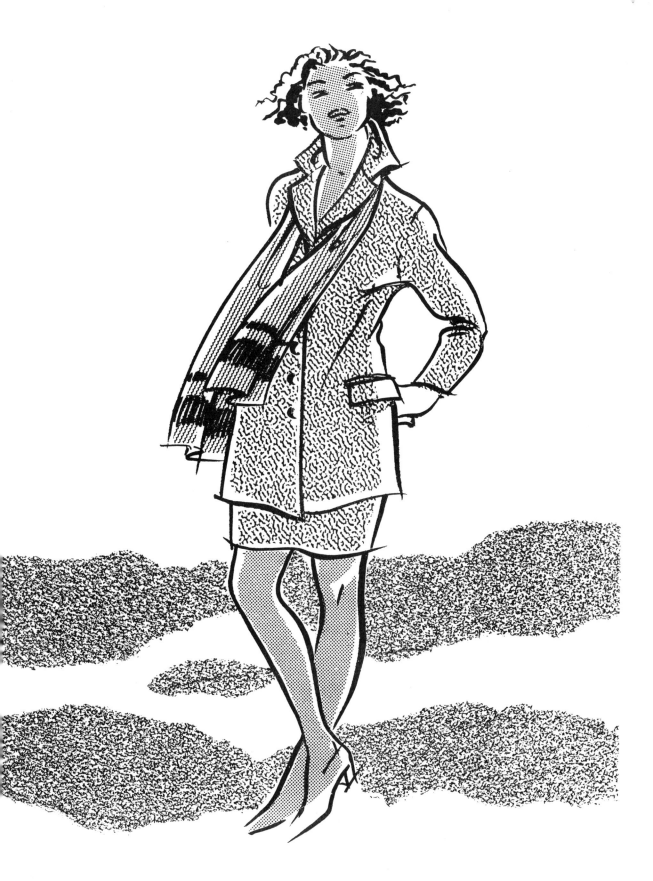

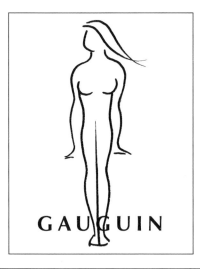

GAUGUIN

Seven-Eighths-Length Jacket Teamed with Leggings

A Perfect Combination for the Gauguin Shape

This jacket also suits the Picasso and Rubens shapes.

■

1. The narrow shawl collar lengthens and slenderizes your upper torso.

2. Dolman sleeves soften square shoulders and give space for a generous bust.

3. The loose jacket in a drapable fabric creates a streamlined silhouette that slenderizes the upper torso.

4. Leggings in a strong accent color highlight slender legs.

5. A monochromatic outfit from head to toe, under open jacket, invites the eye up and down and therefore lengthens and slenderizes your silhouette.

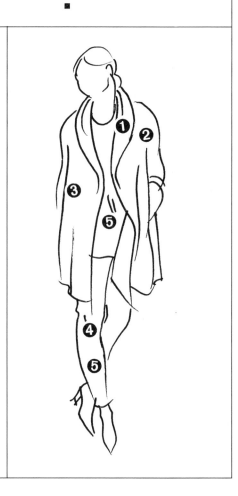

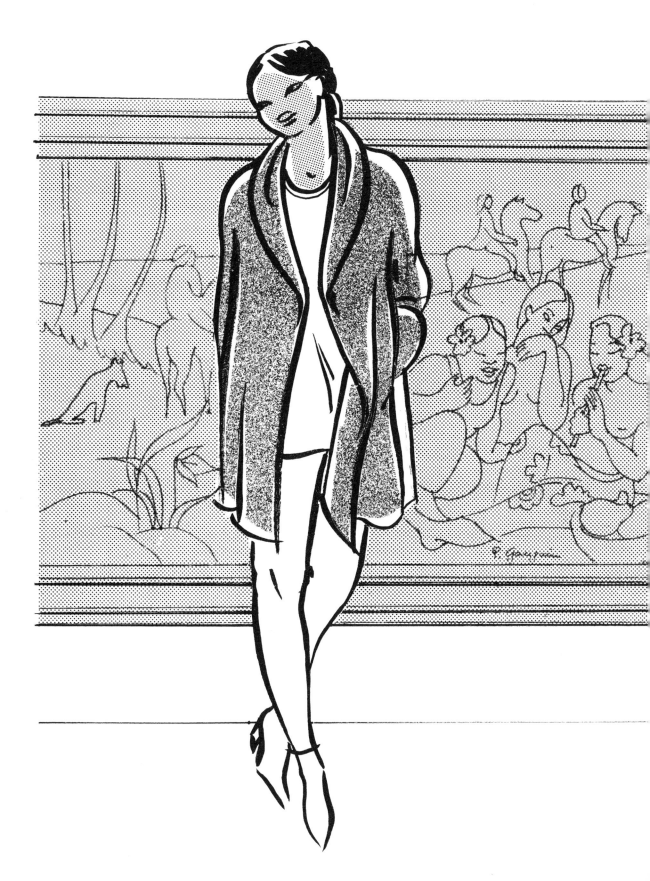

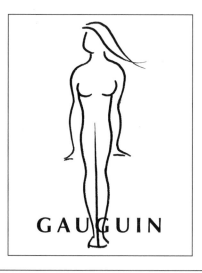

GAUGUIN

Dropped Waist

An Excellent Choice
for the Gauguin Shape

■

1. A deeply colored T-shirt minimizes broad shoulders.

2. The deep V neck slenderizes.

3. Bold, irregular, vertical lines elongate.

4. The dropped waist lengthens and slenderizes the upper torso (avoid if long-waisted).

5. The top is fitted at the hip area to show off your narrow hips.

6. The skirt is gathered to balance your broader upper torso.

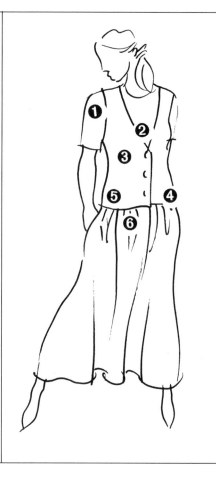

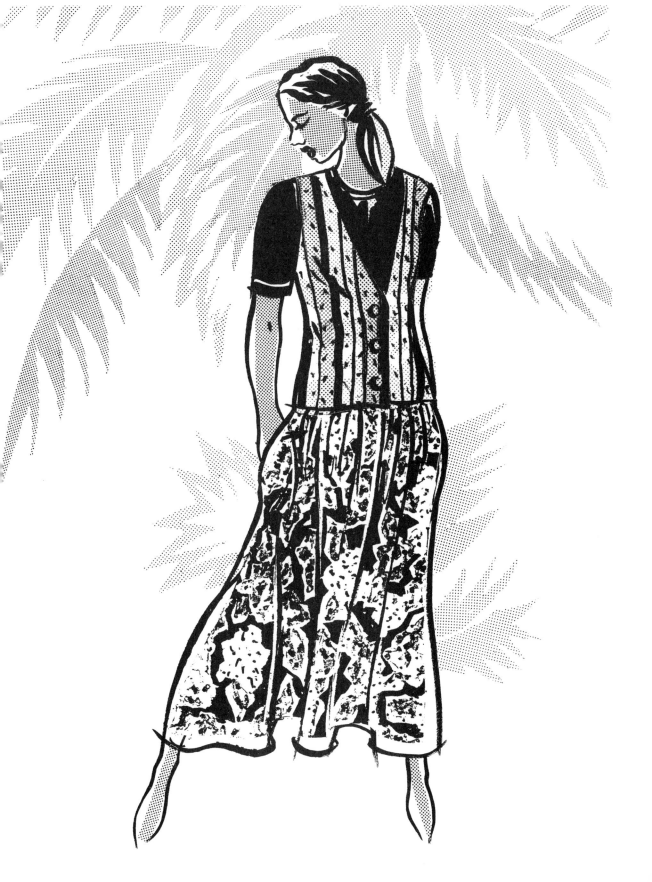

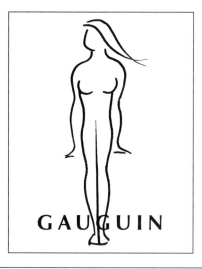

GAUGUIN

Three-Quarters-Length Tunic Teamed with Fluid Palazzo Pants

Creates a Balanced Silhouette for the Gauguin Shape

■

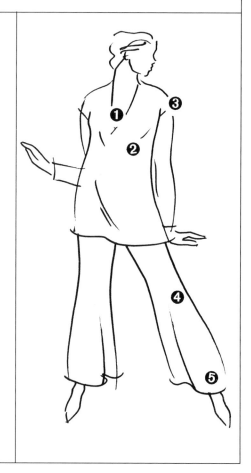

1. The V neck lengthens your neckline.

2. A tunic without details downplays your upper torso.

3. Dropped sleeves (in soft, drapable fabric only) give ease at bust area and soften square shoulders.

4. Large-scaled flower prints invite the eye to your shapely legs (for long legs only).

5. Pants flared at hemline balance broad shoulders (for long legs only).

NOTE: *Palazzo pants should only be worn with high heels.*

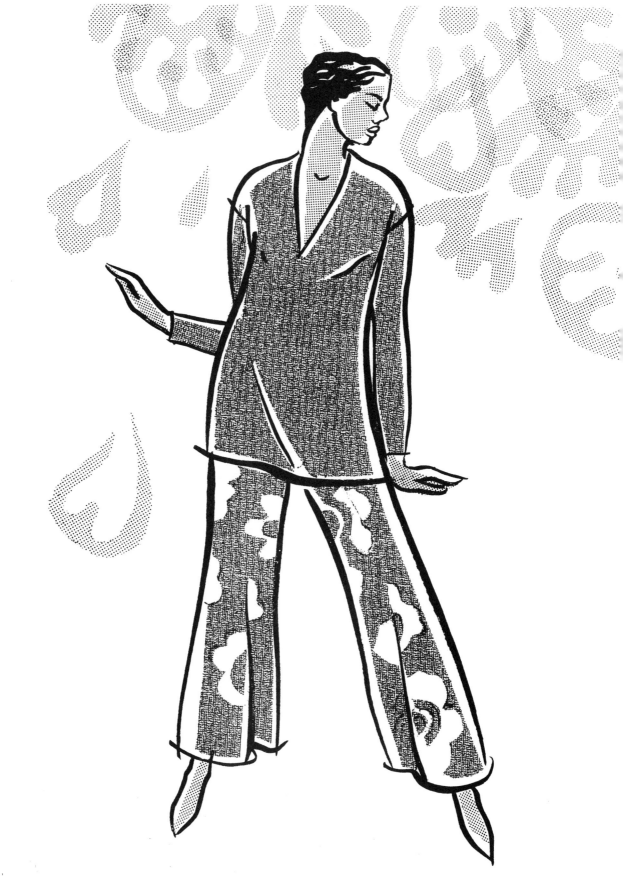

SUMMARY:

Silhouettes that flatter the Gauguin shape minimize your figure challenges, show off your assets, and therefore make you look slimmer.

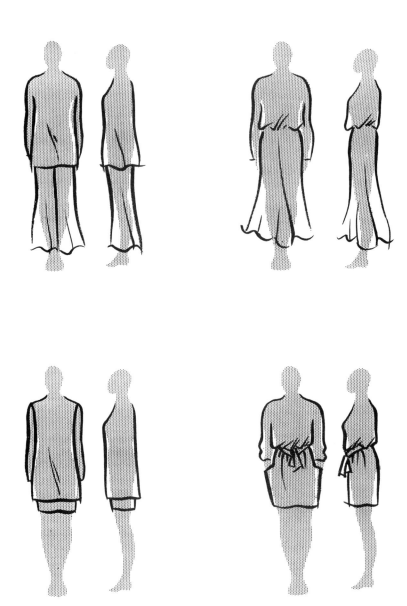

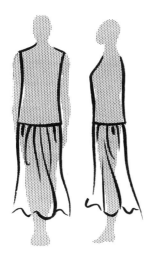
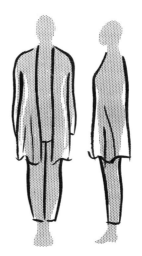

Silhouettes that hide your assets and or expose your figure challenges make you look bigger.

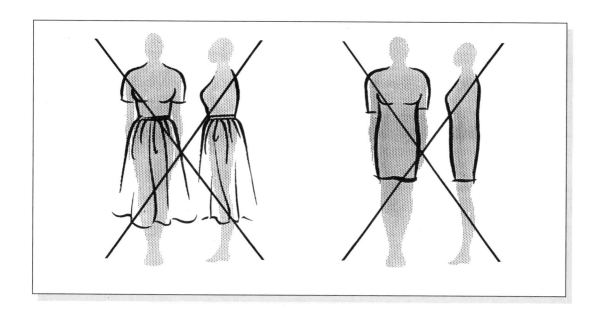

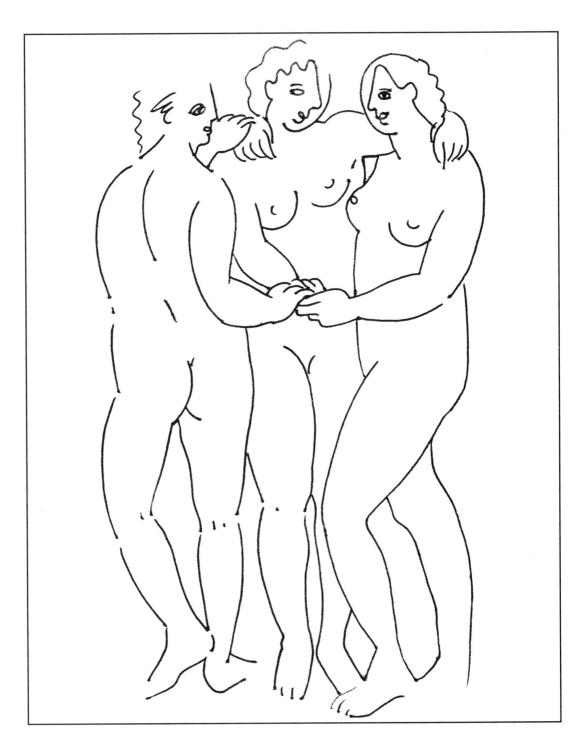

Free interpretation of Picasso's drawing *The Round Dance*.

picasso

Pablo Picasso (1881–1973)

Pablo Ruiz, born in Malaga, Spain, adopted his mother's surname, Picasso, in 1900, at the age of nineteen. His father, who was a painter and a teacher, introduced Pablo to art at an early age and inspired him to pursue studies in La Coruna and Barcelona. In 1904, he established himself in Paris.

During his long life, Picasso has displayed multiple talents in painting, drawing, sculpting, etching, and ceramics. Through his numerous metamorphoses as a painter, he proved to be an artistic pioneer with a central theme: the human being, especially passionate and dramatic women.

When we think of Picasso, we remember his many periods and multiple styles. I have chosen his name to illustrate the straight body shape, referring mainly to his neoclassical period, when he portrayed women with few curves, and his cubist period, where he used straight, angular lines, and cylindrical shapes. If this is you, you are the Picasso type, and you best enhance your body with the same cylindrical shapes and straight, simple lines.

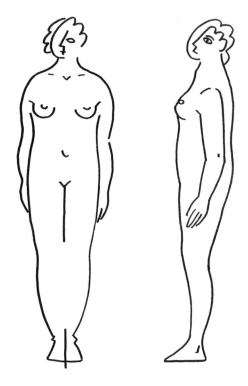

Picasso Shape

CHARACTERISTICS

1. *Upper and lower torso equally wide*

2. Average bust

3. Large rib cage

4. *Undefined waist (often short)*

5. Flat bottom

6. *Slender legs*

To Enhance and Balance Your Silhouette

Slenderize and lengthen your upper torso.

▪

Camouflage your large rib cage.

▪

Deemphasize your waist.

▪

Draw attention to your slender legs.

Picasso (Straight) Shape
General Recommendations

SHAPES AND SILHOUETTES	**Skirts and Pants**	• Just like the Gauguin shape, most skirt syles will suit you, except gathered or tiered skirts, which hide your slender lower hips and thighs. • Skirts without a waistband or with a dropped waistband are the best choice for your undefined waistline. They also visually lengthen your rather short upper torso. • For a comfortable fit and ease at the middle, hips, and thighs, try styles with some Lycra or spandex in the fabric. They fit like a second skin over a full stomach and give additional support. Wear a long top over it to conceal your middle. Same for pants. Skirts or pants that fit your waist are often too wide around your hips. Make sure they have no complicated pockets or topstiching at side seams so that you can taper them easily. • Your best choice are tailored pants in a casual, sporty, or classic, elegant style, such as jeans, hip huggers, stirrups, straight legs and yes, tights, too. All these styles show off your nice legs. But you could also opt for a gentle gathering with an elastic waistband, provided the fabric is fluid enough to drape smoothly over your abdomen. The same style in a stiff or bulky fabric would make you look chunky.
	Tops and Dresses	• Dresses are definitely your best option. Keep them simple and loosely fitted, such as a sheath, a wedge, or a coatdress. The same goes for your jackets and tunics. As your legs are most probably long, you could

SHAPES AND SILHOUETTES (Continued)	**Tops and Dresses** (Continued)	also try dropped waist styles to downplay a missing waist. Tucked-in tops, under an open jacket or cardigan, should always be bloused over your bottom garment to visually lengthen your upper torso. But having your tops float over your middle is an even better choice. The most flattering length for your jackets and tunics are a seven-eighths or a three-quarters length. Even more so, if paired with a short skirt. • Remember! Long compared to short seems even longer. But long, loosely fitting tops require narrow pants or skirts to keep the general look slim. • Please stay away from body-fitting garments. They only emphasize your broad rib cage and not-too-slender waist. The same goes for belted styles. Belts cut your torso horizontally in half and break that desired streamlined effect. • If you are on the short side, make sure that your shoulder pads are not too prominent. Large pads give you a rather stocky, masculine look and make your neck disappear.
COLORS AND PRINTS	**Tops and Bottoms**	• A jacket in a contrasting color should be worn unbuttoned over a shirt, a bodice, or a T-shirt that has the same color as your bottom garment. This creates an unbroken vertical center-front panel. Or wear your tunic or jacket in the same color as your bottom item for a monochromatic outfit. • With your sporty figure, select classic prints such as houndstooth, pinstripes, glen plaids, chevron, geometric patterns, or linear abstracts.

COLORS AND PRINTS (Continued)	**Tops and Bottoms** (Continued)	• Stay clear of small, romantic flower prints; they won't suit your build. • Choose vertical or diagonal prints over your middle. Yes, you can wear medium- to large-scaled prints as long as the color contrast between motif and background is not too bold for your tops. For tall women, a daring, exciting print for skirts and pants make the viewer's eye focus on the bottom half.
FABRICS	**Tops and Bottoms**	• Select your tops in soft, fluid, but nonclingy fabrics for your loosely fitted, generously cut tops. Drapable fabrics will give you a narrow, streamlined silhouette. Your best choices are medium-weight knits, jersey, loose weaves, challis, soft flannels, stonewashed silk, etc. For a straight-line top, opt for a firmer texture, such as linen, gabardine, or tergal. • For your pants and skirts, you can choose any type of fabric, depending upon the style. Fabrics with a low percentage of Lycra or spandex are ideal for you, as they are firm enough for a structured, tailored style without creating those ugly horizontal wrinkles over your stomach, or opt for fluid, drapable fabrics for pants with an elastic waisband to avoid bulk over your abdomen and to provide a narrow, streamlined look (under a long top only).
DETAILS	**Skirts and Pants**	• Here again, keep your bottom items as simple and as classic as possible. If you're tall, you could try some trimmings at the hem level of your skirt to focus attention on your legs. Steer clear of high, tightly fitting waistbands, which shorten and broaden your upper torso and focus attention on your waist.

DETAILS (Continued)	**Tops and Dresses**	• Most lapels and necklines suit your body type. If your neck is on the short side, look for vertical open necklines, such as V or U necks, a notched collar, a tuxedo, or a vertical cowl. • Keep details to a minimum, except for some vertical trimming or edging. Dainty details, such as frills, ruffles, and tiny bows, do not flatter your figure type. Avoid shiny, eye-catching buttons. • Beware of styles with horizontal seams and trimming or piping at midriff, waist, or tummy area.
ACCESSORIES	**Shoes**	• Most designs suit your well-shaped legs. From sporty to elegant, flats or heels, narrow or heavy heels, high-cut or low-cut openings, low boots or high boots, it all works for you. • Avoid overly delicate shoes with fancy details. They look too cute on you.
	Handbags	• Structured, geometric designs will suit a straight figure best. With classic styles, either sporty or elegant, you can't go wrong.
	Belts	• Preferably none! But if you really can't resist, wear one under an open jacket and buckle it loosely enough so the belt falls lower in the front. • Overblouse your tops. • Always keep your belts narrow, and have them blend into the color of your dress or your tops to visually lengthen your upper torso.

ACCESSORIES (Continued)	**Scarves**	• Drape your scarves either loosely around your neck (tightly draped or bulky scarves visually shorten a neck) or have an oblong scarf fall vertically below your abdomen to lengthen your upper torso and invite the eye down to your lower hips. • Stripes, ethnic prints, or abstracts suit you better than a small flower print.
	Jewelry	• Have fun with costume jewelry in simple metal, wood, or plastic. Here again, geometric designs suit you best. • Wear your necklaces either above your middle but below your collarbone, or try long pendants if your abdomen is not too protruding. • For earrings, flat, medium-scaled clusters look best on you. Big hoops or shoulder dusters only look good on women with a long, slender neck, and small studs are better suited for women with a delicate bone structure.

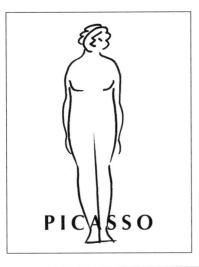

PICASSO

Loosely Fitted Shirtdress

A Timeless Silhouette for the Picasso Shape

This style also suits the Gauguin and Rubens shapes.

■

1. The notch collar provides an open, elongating neckline.

2. The dress is loosely fitted to downplay a missing waist.

3. A single-buttoned front creates vertical interest.

4. The dress is beltless for an unbroken, straight-lined silhouette.

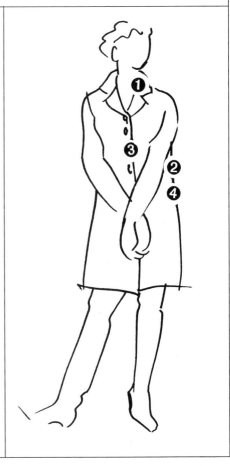

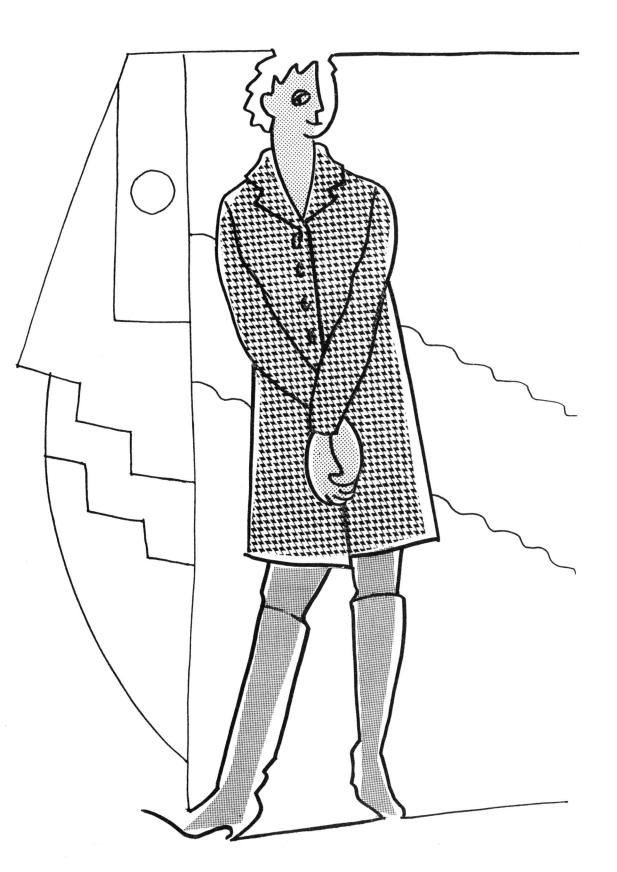

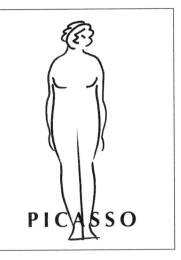

PICASSO

Loosely Fitting Jacket with a Matching Narrow Short Skirt

A Wardrobe Standby for the Picasso Shape

■

1. The V neck provides an open, slenderizing neckline.

2. A necklace that ends below the collarbone elongates the neck.

3. The loosely fitted jacket hides an undefined waist.

4. A three-quarter-length top matched with a short skirt is an ideal proportion to lengthen the upper torso.

5. The single-buttoned top creates vertical center-front interest.

6. Hosiery toned with your skirt gives an elongating look.

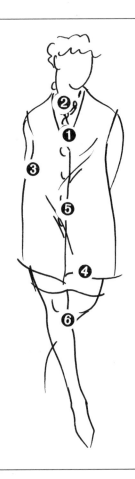

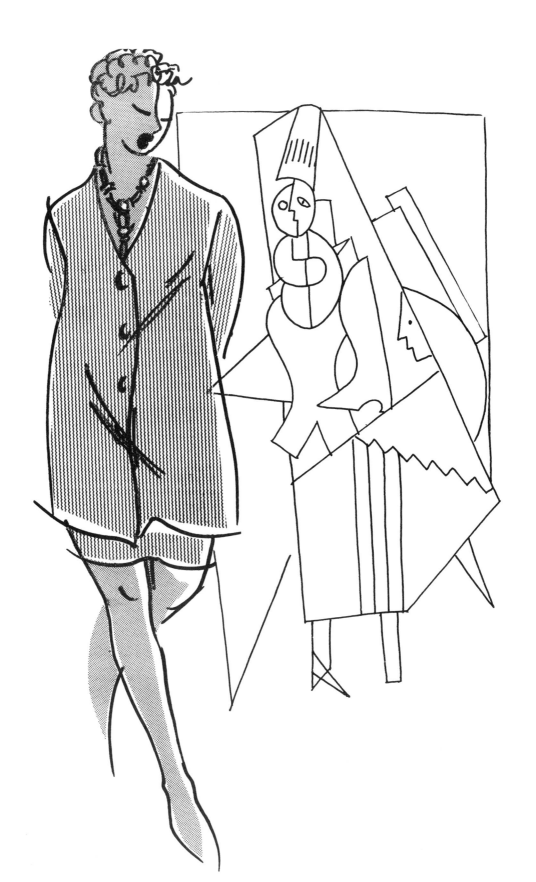

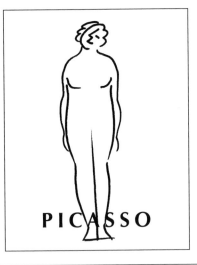

PICASSO

A Shift for Chic Simplicity

A Comfortable and Flattering Silhouette for the Picasso Shape

This style also suits the Gauguin and Rubens shapes.

■

1. The deep V neck lengthens your neckline.

2. The vertical front panels are in two different colors, which elongate.

3. The loose fit camouflages a missing waist.

4. Slit pockets do not break the vertical line of this dress.

5. The side seams of this dress are strategically moved two inches forward from the natural seam position, thereby narrowing the front panels. This gives the illusion of a slimmer silhouette.

6. The dress is softly tapered toward the hemline to create a lean look.

NOTE: This style requires a medium-weight fabric that can be firm or fluid as long as it has enough body to keep the tubular shape of the shift.

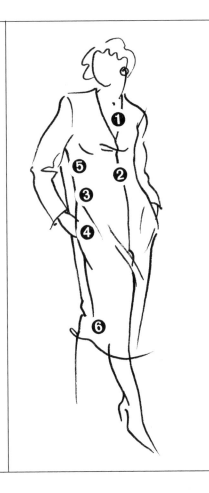

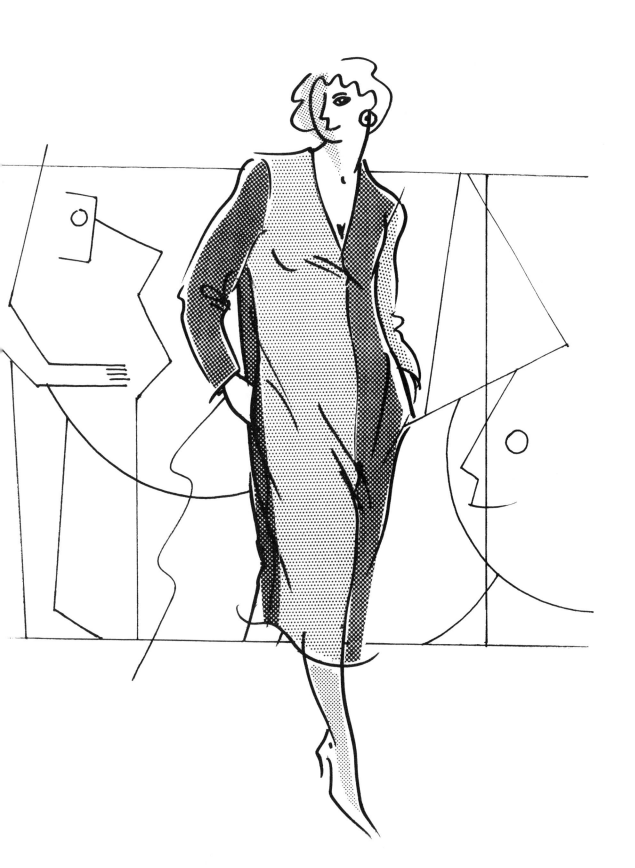

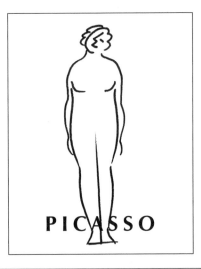

PICASSO

Safari Jacket Teamed with Straight-Leg Pants

A Casual Combination for the Picasso Shape

*This outfit also flatters
the Gauguin shape.*

■

1. The shirt collar standing up at the back visually elongates the neck.

2. The loose fit of the jacket downplays a missing waist.

3. An overbloused T-shirt visually lengthens the upper torso.

4. Narrow, straight pants enhance long legs.

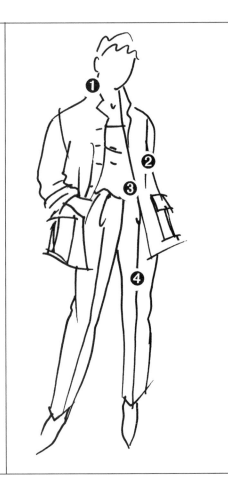

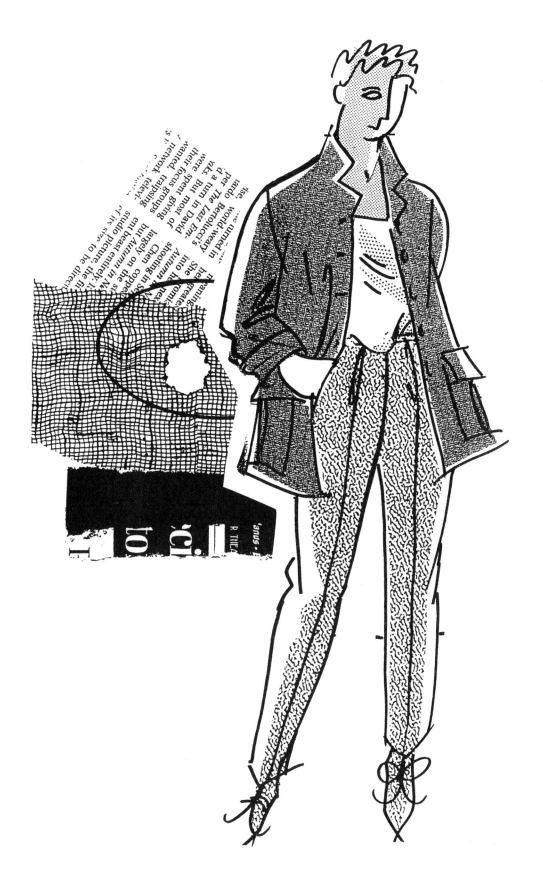

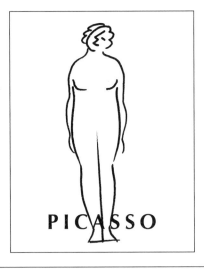

PICASSO

Dropped Waist

An Ideal Silhouette for the Picasso Shape
(If Medium to Tall in Height)

*This style also suits
the Gauguin shape.*

■

1. The dropped waist elongates and slenderizes the upper torso.

2. No details at the bustline downplay that area.

3. The skirt is slightly gathered, in a drapable fabric only, to keep the silhouette streamlined and narrow.

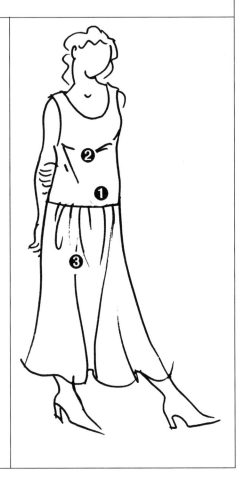

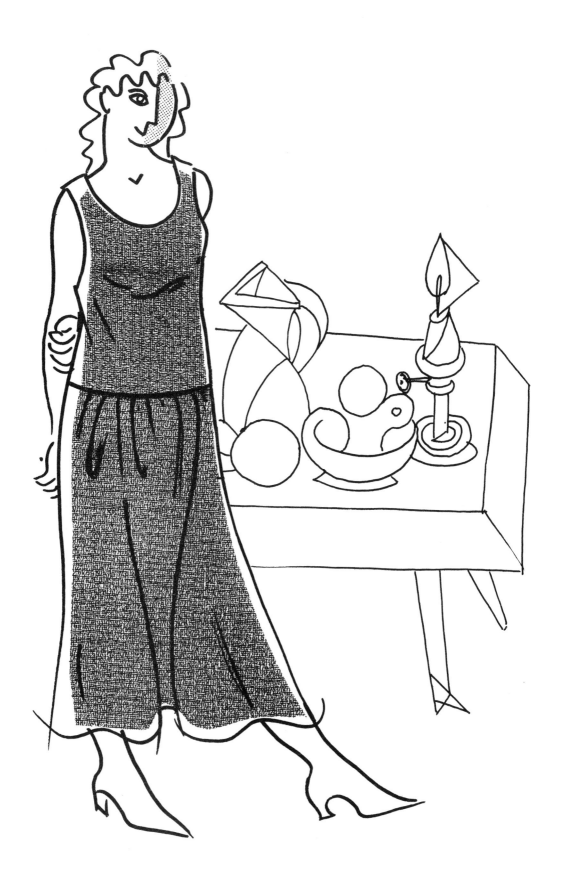

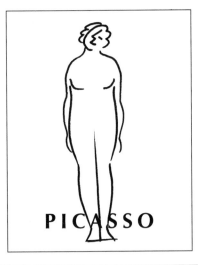

PICASSO

Tunic Dress for the Picasso Shape

A Flattering Silhouette for the Evening

This style also suits the Rubens and Gauguin shapes.

∎

1. Cluster earrings suit a short neck best.

2. A neckline below the collarbone elongates your neck.

3. A sheer top over a deeply colored, slimming base enhances most figures and gives a feminine touch to the Picasso shape.

4. The vertical pattern on tulle has a lengthening effect.

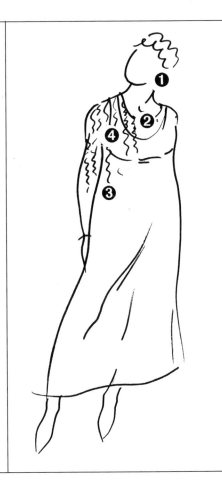

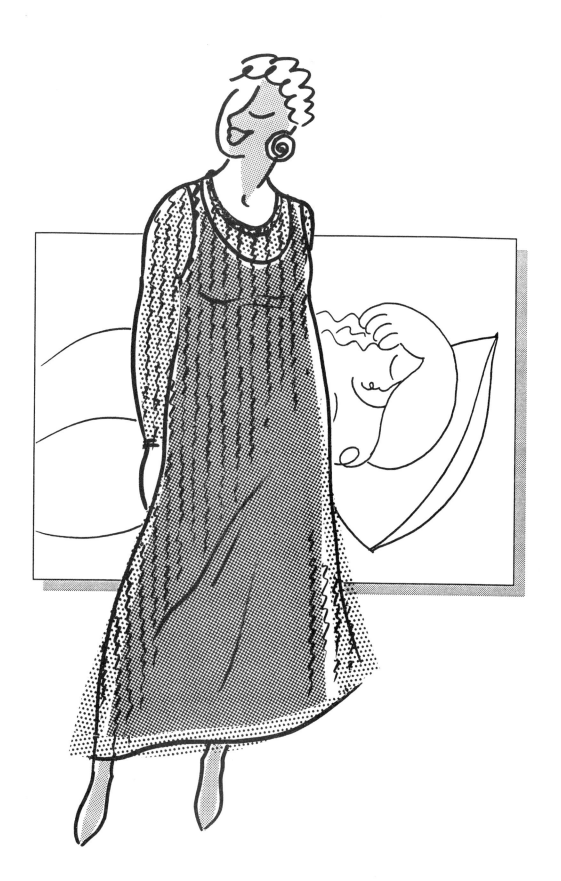

SUMMARY:

Silhouettes that flatter the Picasso shape minimize your figure challenges, show off your assets, and therefore make you look slimmer.

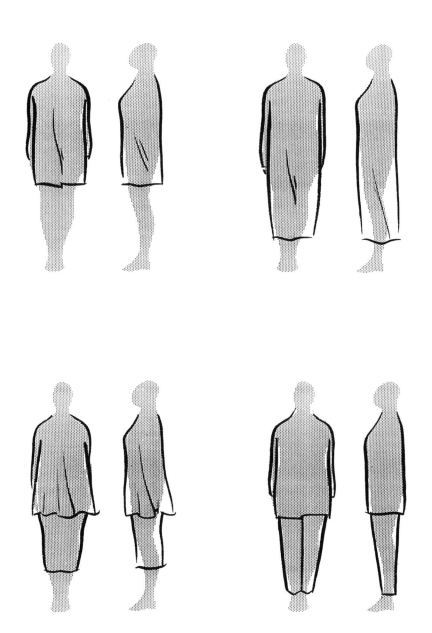

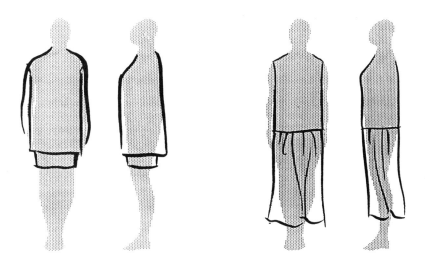

Silhouettes that hide your assets or expose your figure challenges make you look bigger.

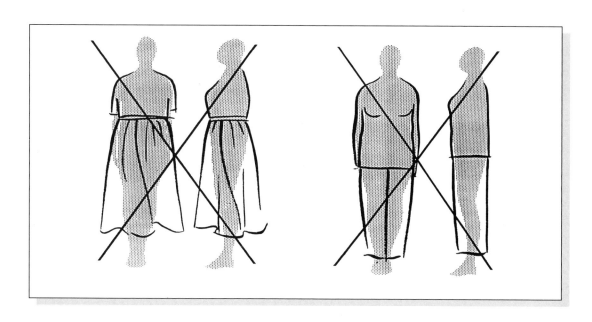

summary charts

recommended items according

to various body shapes

SKIRTS

TYPE OF SKIRT / BODY TYPE	Tailored *Firm Fabric or Lycra*	Slightly Gathered *Drapey Fabric*	Straight, Gently Gathered	Straight, Tailored *Firm Fabric*	Knife Pleats *Lightweight, Soft, or Knit*
modigliani	★ (2)(3)(4)	★★★ (4)	★★★	★★ (2)(3)	★ (2)
renoir	✕	✕	★★★ (2)	★ (2)	★★ (2)
rubens	★ (2)(4)	★★ (2)(4)	★★★ (2)	★★ (2)	★★★ (2)
pop art	★★ (4)	★★★ (4)	★★★	★★	✕
gauguin	★★★	★★	★ (2)	★★★ (2)	★★★ (2)
picasso	★★ (2)(4)	★★★ (4)	★★ (2)	★★	★★ (2)

★★★   YOUR VERY BEST CHOICE

★★   FLATTERING

★   OK

✕   TO AVOID

(1) If medium to tall in height

(2) Teamed with a long top

(3) Teamed with a hipbone-length top

(4) Only for shapely legs

SKIRTS (Continued)

TYPE OF SKIRT / BODY TYPE	Wrapped or Sarong *Drapey Fabric*	Trumpet *Firm or Drapey*	Tulip *Firm Fabric*	Flared *Drapey Fabric*	A-line *Firm Fabric*
modigliani	★★★	✕	★	★★★ (3)	★
renoir	★	✕	✕	✕	✕
rubens	✕	★ (2)(1)	✕	✕	✕
pop art	★★★	★ (1)	★★	★★	★ (1)
gauguin	★★	★★★ (1)	★	★★★ (2)	★★ (1)
picasso	★ (4)	★★ (2)(1)	✕	★	✕

★★★ YOUR VERY BEST CHOICE
★★ FLATTERING
★ OK
✕ TO AVOID

(1) If medium to tall in height
(2) Teamed with a long top
(3) Teamed with a hipbone-length top
(4) Only for shapely legs

SKIRTS (Continued)

TYPE OF SKIRT / BODY TYPE	Pleats, Top-Stiched up to Hipbone *Firm Fabric*	Hip Yoke, Gathered *Drapey Fabric*	Circular *Drapey Fabric*	Tiered *Firm or Drapey Fabric*	Full Skirt (Dirndl) *Firm or Drapey Fabric*
modigliani	✕	✕	✕	✕	✕
renoir	✕	✕	✕	✕	✕
rubens	✕	✕	✕	✕	✕
pop art	★	★	★★ (1)	★★ (1)	★★
gauguin	★★	★★★ (1)	★	★ (1)	✕
picasso	★ (2)	✕	✕	✕	✕

★★★ Your Very Best Choice

★★ Flattering

★ OK

✕ To Avoid

(1) If medium to tall in height

(2) Teamed with a long top

(3) Teamed with a hipbone-length top

(4) Only for shapely legs

PANTS

TYPE OF PANTS / BODY TYPE	Leggings *Stretch Fiber or Knit*	Bell-bottoms *Drapey or Firm Fabric*	Jeans, Semifitted *Stretch or Firm Fabric*	Straight Leg, Tailored *Firm Fabric*	Stirrup *Firm, with Stretch Fiber*
modigliani	✕	✕	★	✕	★
renoir	✕	✕	✕	✕ (2)	★ (2)
rubens	★ (2)	✕	★ (2)	★ (2)	★★★ (2)
pop art	★	★ (1)	★★	✕	★★
gauguin	★★ (2)	★★ (1)	★★★	★★★	★★
picasso	★★ (2)	✕	★★★ (2)	★★★ (2)	★★ (2)

★★★ YOUR VERY BEST CHOICE
 ★★ FLATTERING
  ★ OK
  ✕ TO AVOID

(1) If medium to tall in height
(2) Teamed with a long top
(3) Drapable fabric only
(4) Not to be worn by itself

PANTS (Continued)

TYPE OF PANTS / BODY TYPE	Elasticized Pants, Loosely Fitted, Tapered at Hem Level	Wide, Straight Leg *Firm or Drapey Fabric*	Bermuda Shorts *Firm Fabric*	Cuffed Shorts *Firm Fabric*	Hot Pants *Firm Fabric*
modigliani	★★★	★ (1)	✕	✕	✕
renoir	★★★	✕	✕	✕	✕
rubens	★★ (2)(4)	★ (1)	★ (2)	✕	✕
pop art	★★	★ (1)	★★	✕	★★
gauguin	✕	★ (1)	★★	★★	★★
picasso	★★ (2)(4)	★ (1)	★★ (2)	★★	✕

★★★ YOUR VERY BEST CHOICE
★★ FLATTERING
★ OK
✕ TO AVOID

(1) If medium to tall in height
(2) Teamed with a long top
(3) Drapable fabric only
(4) Not to be worn by itself

PANTS (Continued)

TYPE OF PANTS / BODY TYPE	Elasticized Shorts *Drapey Fabric*	Culottes *Firm Fabric*	Culottes *Drapey Fabric*	Palazzo Pants *Drapey Fabric*	Harem Pants *Drapey Fabric*
modigliani	★★	✕	★★	★ (1)	★ (1)
renoir	★	✕	★★★ (2)	✕	✕
rubens	★★ (2)	✕	★★ (2)	★ (1)	✕
pop art	★★★	✕	★★	★ (1)	★ (1)
gauguin	★★	★ (1)	★★	★ (1)	★★ (1)
picasso	★★ (2)	★	★★ (2)	★ (3)	✕

★★★   YOUR VERY BEST CHOICE   (1) If medium to tall in height
 ★★   FLATTERING   (2) Teamed with a long top
  ★   OK   (3) Drapable fabric only
  ✕   TO AVOID   (4) Not to be worn by itself

TOPS

TYPE OF TOP / BODY TYPE	Tank Top, Body Contoured *Knit or Stretch*	T-shirt, Softly Waisted *Knit*	Basque, Fitted *Firm Fabric*	Short, Bloused *Knit*	Cropped Top *Firm Fabric*
modigliani	★	★★★ (3)	★	★★	★★★
renoir	✕	✕	✕	✕	★
rubens	✕	✕	✕	✕	✕
pop art	★ (3)	★★★ (3)	★★★ (5)	★★★	★
gauguin	✕	★★	✕	★★	✕
picasso	✕	✕	✕	★	✕

★★★ YOUR VERY BEST CHOICE

★★ FLATTERING

★ OK

✕ TO AVOID

(1) If medium to tall in height
(2) Teamed with a narrow skirt
(3) Only in soft, drapable fabric
(4) Worn unbuttoned
(5) If your curves are not too voluptuous

TOPS (Continued)

TYPE OF TOP → / BODY TYPE ↓	Cardigan, Slightly Fitted *Drapey or Firm Fabric*	Chanel Jacket, Boxy *Drapey or Firm Fabric*	Belted Safari Jacket, Overbloused *Firm Fabric*	Blazer, Straight *Firm or Drapey Fabric*	Overshirt *Firm or Drapey Fabric*
modigliani	★★★	★ (4)	★	★ (4)	★ (4)
renoir	★	✕	✕	★	★
rubens	✕	✕	✕	★★	★★
pop art	★★★	★ (4)	★★★ (5)	✕	★ (4)
gauguin	★ (3)	★	★★	★★	★★
picasso	✕	✕	✕	★★★	★★★

★★★ YOUR VERY BEST CHOICE
★★ FLATTERING
★ OK
✕ TO AVOID

(1) If medium to tall in height
(2) Teamed with a narrow skirt
(3) Only in soft, drapable fabric
(4) Worn unbuttoned
(5) If your curves are not too voluptuous

TOPS (Continued)

TYPE OF TOP BODY TYPE	Suit Jacket, Fitted *Firm Fabric*	Jacket, Loosely Fitted, Double-Breasted *Firm Fabric*	Tunic, Loosely Fitted *Drapey Fabric*	Cardigan, Loosely Fitted *Drapey Fabric*	Tunic, Flared *Drapey Fabric*
modigliani	✕	✕	✕	★ (4)	✕
renoir	✕	★	★	★ (4)	★★ (1) (3)
rubens	✕	★	★★★ (2)(3)	★★ (4)	★★ (1)(2)(3)
pop art	★★ (5)	✕	✕	✕	✕
gauguin	✕	★★	★★★ (2)(3)	★★★ (2)	★★ (1)(2)(3)
picasso	✕	★★	★★★ (2)(3)	★★★ (2)(3)	★★ (1)(2)(3)

★★★ YOUR VERY BEST CHOICE
★★ FLATTERING
★ OK
✕ TO AVOID

(1) If medium to tall in height
(2) Teamed with a narrow skirt
(3) Only in soft, drapable fabric
(4) Worn unbuttoned
(5) If your curves are not too voluptuous

DRESSES

TYPE OF DRESS / BODY TYPE	Tank Dress, Body Contoured *Knit*	Shift, Semifitted *Drapey Fabric*	Shift, Straight *Drapey or Firm Fabric*	Shift, Belted, Overbloused	Shift with Loosely Fitted Sash *Drapey Fabric*
modigliani	✕	★★	✕	★ (1)	✕
renoir	✕	✕	✕	✕	✕
rubens	✕	✕	★★	✕	★ (1)
pop art	★★	★★★	✕	★★ (1)	★
gauguin	✕	★★	★★	★★	★★★ (1)
picasso	✕	✕	★★★	✕	★★ (1)

★★★   Your Very Best Choice   (1) If medium to tall in height

★★   Flattering

★   OK

✕   To Avoid

DRESSES (Continued)

TYPE OF DRESS → BODY TYPE ↓	Dropped Waist *Drapey Fabric*	Slightly Dropped Waist *Drapey Fabric*	Empire Dress Fitted Over Bust *Drapey Fabric Only*	Empire Dress Fitted Over Bust, Gathered *Drapey Fabric*	Surplice or Wrap Dress *Drapey Fabric Only*
modigliani	✕	★	★★★	★★	★★
renoir	✕	★ (1)	★	★★★	★★
rubens	✕	✕	✕	✕	★
pop art	✕	✕	★	✕	★★★
gauguin	★★★ (1)	★ (1)	★	✕	★
picasso	★★ (1)	★ (1)	✕	✕	★

★★★   YOUR VERY BEST CHOICE   (1) If medium to tall in height

★★   FLATTERING

★   OK

✕   TO AVOID

DRESSES (Continued)

TYPE OF DRESS → BODY TYPE ↓	Coat Dress, Straight *Firm Fabric*	Coat Dress, Semifitted *Firm Fabric*	Tent or Trapeze Dress *Drapey Fabric*	Wedge Dress *Drapey Fabric Only*	A-line, Semifitted *Drapey Fabric*
modigliani	✕	★	✕	✕	★
renoir	✕	✕	★★★	★★	✕
rubens	★★★	✕	★★	★★★	✕
pop art	✕	★★	✕	✕	★★
gauguin	★★★	★	✕	★★ (1)	★
picasso	★★★	★	★	★★★	✕

★★★   YOUR VERY BEST CHOICE   (1) If medium to tall in height
  ★★   FLATTERING
   ★   OK
   ✕   TO AVOID

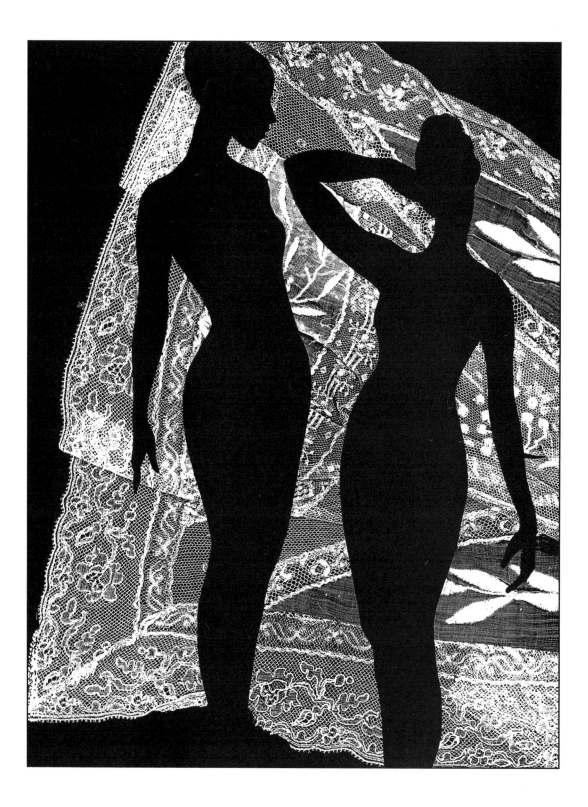

particulars

UNDERWEAR

Selecting the appropriate underwear for your body shape should be taken as seriously as choosing the right outerwear. Perfectly fitting lingerie contributes to the general appearance of your silhouette and is an integral part of the "dressing slim" strategy. Quality underwear may cost more, but the benefits are worth it. Good underwear not only allows your clothes to fit to their best advantage, but it also makes you feel terrific. Treat yourself! It's an affordable luxury.

Brassieres

General Recommendations

Different fabrics, décolletés, and designs of your garments require different bra styles. Each brand of underwear has its own variety of styles and sizes, so don't hesitate to ask for professional advice. A competent salesperson will know which brand, structure, design, and size will suit you best and therefore help you to save time, hassle, and money. **A bra that gives an unflattering shape to your bustline can ruin the most expensive outfit, whereas the right bra will support your bust and give you the most flattering shape possible.** Make sure to have at least one or two skin-tone-colored bras, which are an absolute must under semi- or fully transparent clothes. The same goes for panties, slips, and camisoles. The bare color should be slightly darker than your skin, so it won't show through. When you wear a sleeveless top, always make sure that the armhole covers your bra. A bra showing under the arm always looks sloppy.

Small Bust

If your cup size is A or B, you have a small bust. Don't be troubled about your bust size. Rather, consider yourself lucky. A small bust holds up by itself. Besides, a sexy bust is a question of shape, not size. However, if you do want a little extra to balance a heavier bottom half, look for filled contour bras, slightly padded bras, push-ups, or bras with shapes molded into the cup. They are the best solution for dresses with a deep neckline. Avoid bras with seams that cross the nipples. Choose seamless bras under semifitting bodies or lightweight fabrics for a more natural look. Bras with reinforced side panels will press your breasts toward the middle, which will create the desired illusion of cleavage and a fuller bustline.

Large Bust

For really heavy breasts, wired cups provide the best shape and support. Unfortunately, because of the wiring, they can be rather uncomfortable to wear all day long, so make sure that the wiring is flat and well padded. Shoulder straps carry your breasts, so select styles with wide enough straps to cut the pressure on the shoulder. Elasticized straps overstretch easily. Look for adjustable ones or replace them once they are worn out, but only if the rest of the bra is still in perfect condition. Worn-out, overstretched bras won't give you the support you need and therefore would make your bust sag. A bra has to support, shape, and lift your breast. By *lift*, I don't mean you should push your breasts upward to an unnatural height. A good height is one inch below the midpoint between shoulder and waist. Everything above is unnatural and would just make your breasts bulge out over the top and give the illusion of having two pairs of breasts, one on top of the other! Cups that are too small would cause the same effect and make your breasts look bigger than they actually are. Avoid those ghastly bulges caused by bras that fit too tightly around the body.

Jiggling and bouncing of the breasts can be embarassing and painful. Consider wearing a minimizer or a sport bra. These styles give you support and comfort without hindering your movements. When trying on a sport bra for active sports, jump and move to make sure you get all the suport you need for your breast. Some women prefer the strong, highly elasticized, compression type of bra, which keeps the breasts tight to the body and feel comfortable enough for everyday wear. As it does not really shape or lift your breast, you should wear this type of bra under loosely fitting tops only. You will also find another style of sport bra that separates your breast better; it has separate cups on the inside with additional elastic strap control in Lycra at the outer side of the cups.

Short-waisted women are better off with cup-style bras or cups with underwire support, as these styles separate the bust from the waist better and give more space to the upper torso.

Camisoles and Slips

Always wear a slip or camisole under your clothes. It helps your garments drape better over your curves and prevents them from clinging. It also acts as a lining to hide a panty line or lumps and bulges caused by tight bras, panties, or girdles. Besides, it is a pleasure to feel those silky-smooth textures on your skin. A good trick to prevent a top from clinging to your pants or skirts is to wear your camisole over your bottom items (if your top is long enough) instead of tucking them in. This will also camouflage any bulge of a protruding stomach, caused by tight waistbands, especially under transparent or lightweight fabrics. A slip will help a flared skirt drape better, reveal less of your hips and thighs under a narrow skirt, and prevent your skirt from bagging. When you wear a long top over your skirt, wear a camisole under your top and, yes, a slip under your skirt. This will make the cheapest outfit fall better and make it look so much more chic.

Panties

For small buttocks, the choice in design and fabrics are endless. If you're bottom-heavy, forget about tiny bikini panties under tightly fitted pants or skirts. The panty line would show for sure. Panties under fitted clothes should cover your entire bottom and tummy and end either at the waist or just one inch below. Shorts-style panties are pretty and comfortable under loose skirts and pants, but they create wrinkles under snug-fitting clothes.

Body Shapers and Control Panties

Don't wear anything that you find uncomfortable just for the sake of looking slimmer. But many women do not have a problem with control panties. They come in blends of Lycra and microfibers, are light, and won't restrict your digestion or keep you from breathing properly, while still giving you some control.

Keep body shapers with a high percentage of stretch fibers for special, dressy occasions only. Beware of excessively tight hosieries, girdles, or control panties, as they would provoke bulges at waist and thighs. *If you need a girdle, avoid snug-fitting clothes.*

If your thighs need slimming, opt for panties or hosieries with special thigh support. To prevent a thigh rash, slide panty liners inside your hose or panties at the inner thighs, just where your thighs rub togethr. The adhesive will keep them in place.

Colors

As far as colors are concerned, you just need white or ivory-colored lingerie to wear under light-colored clothes, black to wear under dark colors, and skin-toned lingerie to wear under fully or semitransparent clothes. The bare color of your underwear should be slightly darker than your skin.

SWIMSUITS

General Recommendations

Take your time when shopping for a swimsuit. Your first criterion should be comfort, and comfort means a perfect fit. Don't go for less than perfect, as alterations are not possible. You may feel safe with a designer label you're familiar with, as many designers and manufacturers are quite consistent in design, size, and structure. But try it on, nonetheless.

Again, choose a design that flatters your body shape. Don't be shy to take advice from a qualified salesperson and an honest friend with a critical eye, for a more objective opinion.

For colors, details, and proportions, apply the same principles as outlined for clothes (see the chart for your particular body type in chapter 8). Remember, use dark colors to cover your challenges and light colors to expose your assets and to divert attention from your weak points. Colors wisely placed can reshape and balance your figure. Black is the most receding color to minimize any curve or bulge, but it can look a bit harsh on white skin. Some edging in a bright color at the neckline will soften the contrast. Many bathing suits have a shiny texture. Beware of this if you are on the heavy side; they reveal each little bulge and overemphasize your curves. They only look great on a perfect figure.

The fabric of your bathing suit should be stretchy but firm to shape your figure. The difference in stretch and flexibility depends on the percentage of spandex, Lycra, or other stretch fibers in the fabric. Most are blends of stretch and microfibers. These new textures are light, comfortable, and they dry quickly. There are many different blends, and their stretchability and firmness varies from one suit to the other. Therefore, always try on a bathing suit before buying. A suit that is too firm or excessively elasticized might be uncomfortable for you but just right for somebody else, and a fabric with a very low percentage of stretchy yarn may give you enough support but may not be firm enough for someone else.

Recommendations According to
Your Body Shape

Modigliani

- Consider styles with a focus point at bust level to bring the eye up, away from your challenges.

- Favour strapless styles that will create strong horizontal lines and visually widen your bustline and balance your bottom half.

- Darker side panels will take a few inches away from your hips. Select high-cut leg openings in the front only, but make sure your rear is covered.

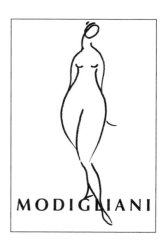

Renoir

- The same guidelines as outlined in the Modigliani chapter are also recommended for your body shape.

- Wrapped or skirted styles are the answer for really heavy thighs or a big stomach.

- Sometimes a simple one-piece swimsuit in a deep color over your challenges, with an exciting touch of color or design detail at bust level, is a good enough trick to divert attention from your bottom half.

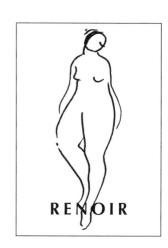

Rubens

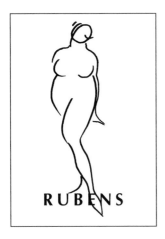

- For your bustline, refer to the recommendations as outlined in the Gauguin shape.

- To keep a protruding stomach in place, consider wearing a swimsuit with an inside control panel. These elastic panels are light but firm enough to give your stomach the support it needs. Another key to the problem is to wear skirted, wrapped or overbloused styles. I, myself, recommend the use of the color strategy (see #2 in General Recommendations). That really works wonders in minimizing and balancing challenges. Diagonal styles or prints over the stomach help to downplay that area.

Pop Art

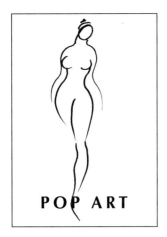

- Bikini? A one-piece swimsuit? You look great in both. If your curves are on the Baroque side, opt for wrapped or surplice styles. Just make sure to choose styles that are structured in such a way to carry the weight of your impressive bustline. Halter-neck styles highlight your curved shoulders, provide a nice cleavage and suit your feminine body shape.

Gauguin

- U- or V-neck décolletés will visually lengthen your upper torso. Avoid horizontal necklines, as this would just emphasize your broad shoulders. Beware of a halter-neck top for the same reason. If your bust is really ample, look for designs with formed cups. Make sure that they are large enough, so that your bust won't come out at the top. If you feel uncomfortable with underwiring, do consider other solutions to keep your bust in place, such as inner panels or specially structured designs which keep the breast tight to the body, to avoid jiggling or boucing of the bust. Select styles with armholes that do not gape, so your bust won't slip out at the side. That would give your bust an unflattering form.

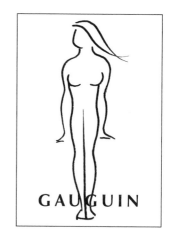

Picasso

- With your not-too-defined (often short) torso, you definitely look best in a one-piece swimsuit. To define your waist, select styles with darker side panels. It is the best solution for a missing waist. If these side panels widen toward waist level, it reinforces the slimming effect even more.

- Another trick to visually slenderize your waist is to create a strong vertical center interest to help the eye move up and down and draw attention toward the center and away from the side. Choose styles with vertical seams or prints to visually elongate an upper torso.

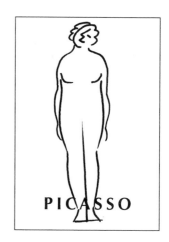

Examples

Modigliani

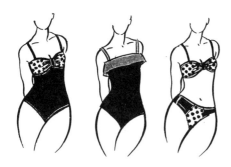

Left: Toned-down colors at the bottom downplay your challenge. Strong, loud, contrasting colors at bust level divert attention from your bottom half.

Center: A bright panel creates a strong horizontal line, visually widens this area, and balances heavy hips.

Right: The design of this bikini bottom leads the eye to the center, away from your hips. Along with the dark side panels, it maximizes the slimming effect. A high-cut leg opening visually lengthens and slenderizes the legs. This bikini top will enlarge a small bust.

Renoir

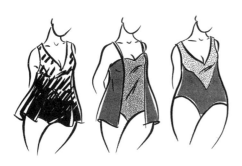

Left: The gradually wider-spaced print lightens toward the bust area. Therefore, it brings the eye up and diverts attention from your weak points. The skirted swimsuit will cover ample hips and upper thighs.

Center: This swimsuit with darker side panels, which finishes as a skirt at the sides and back, is the best solution to conceal voluptuous hips, thighs, and rear and to provide ease in that area.

Right: This swimsuit is a good example of a perfect color strategy. The lighter color at the top will bring the eye up, away from your challenges. The diagonal seams at the front deemphasize a big stomach area.

Rubens

Left: Diagonals slenderize.

Center: This surplice style gives enough ease at stomach area. The asymmetric design creates an interest point at the top. The V-neck opening is a perfect neckline for a rather padded neck.

Right: The skirted style conceals an ample stomach and gives you ease where you need it. Vertical panels slenderize.

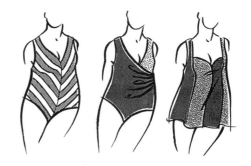

Pop Art

Left: This halter top gives you ease at the bust area and prevents your bust from flattening out toward the side.

Center: A one-piece swimsuit with an inside cup in a solid color shows off your perfect figure. A double or triple string, which wraps loosely around your waist, helps to focus attention to your terrific waistline.

Right: A bikini top for a more voluptuous bustline. Cups with underwiring and side panels that end in a halter neck help to carry the weight of your bust.

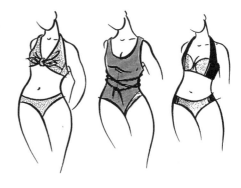

Gauguin

Left: Gradual shading from dark at the top to light at the bottom creates vertical interest. The deeper colors at the bust level visually minimize that area. The bigger the contrast, the greater the effect.

Center: The side panel ending as a shoulder strap carries the weight of your bust and prevents the bust slipping out at the side.

Right: Vertical all-over prints invite the eye up and down and deemphasize the bust.

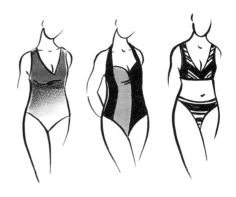

Picasso

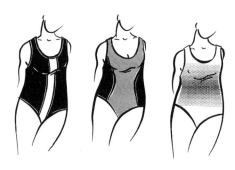

Left: A narrow vertical front panel in a bright, contrasting color leads the eye up and down and helps to focus attention to the center and thereby slenderize.

Center: Dark side panels that get larger at waist level are the most efficient tricks to slenderize a waistline.

Right: Gradually shading from light to dark, with the darkest color at the waistline deemphasizes that area.

problem areas

SHORT AND/OR HEAVY NECK

- Your neck will look longer and thinner if you keep your neckline **open**.

- Unbutton the first few buttons of a tightly fitting neckline.

- Collars should be narrow. Have them stand up behind the neck to reinforce the V neckline effect.

- V neck openings are your best bet. A crew neckline, which chokes you, will only accentuate your challenge. Other options: U neckline, sweetheart, or deep décolletés.

- Don't try to hide your neck with bulky scarves. It would make your neck look even shorter. Select oblong scarves rather than squares ones. The texture should be fine and drapable. Let them hang loose or knot or drape them low. This will visually add more length to your neck.

- Stay away from bold or heavy earrings, especially long ones such as big hoops, drops, or shoulder dusters, as those would actually make a neck look even shorter. Flat, medium-scaled clusters will look best on you.

- Chokers are very unflattering. They horizontally divide an already short neck and focus attention to that area.

- Pendants, strings of beads, or pearls that end below the collarbone are a better choice for a short neck.

- In the cold season, you might feel like covering your neck. Opt for vertical cowls rather than tightly fitted and/or bulky turtlenecks. Add a loose-hanging, oblong scarf to create vertical lines. This will also counter the effect of a covered neck.

- Avoid too much hair at neck area, as this would make your neck appear shorter. A short, feminine, layered hairstyle, maybe pointed toward the back of your neck, or any pinned-up style will lengthen your neck.

- Stay clear of large shoulder pads! They will lift your shoulders and make your already short neck disappear. The same goes for epaulettes.

NARROW AND/OR SLOPING SHOULDERS

- Narrow shoulders that are in proportion with the rest of your body are not a challenge. But if your shoulders are narrower than your bottom half, you need shoulder pads for a more balanced appearance. The same goes for sloping shoulders, but beware of pads that are too big, especially if you are short. Look for the size that is best for your body to achieve a balanced proportion.

- Round shoulders curve forward and seem to be narrower than they actually are. A good trick to straighten round shoulders is to slip your pads a tiny bit toward the back and have the blunt edge of your pads exceed your shoulder bones by a half inch.

- Use only skin-toned pads for transparent, thin, or white clothes.

- Prefer structured, tailored styles to unstructured, droopy styles. Set-in sleeves, placed slightly outside your shoulder bones, work wonders. Take the next size up for your top, and have it tapered in at bust level.

- Halter necklines visually widen narrow shoulders, but avoid them if your shoulders are sloping.

For more details, see your chart in chapter 8.

BROAD SHOULDERS

Large shoulders are only an issue if they are not in proportion to your bottom half. If your bottom half is narrow in contrast to your broad shoulders, follow these guidelines.

- Large shoulders allow your garments to fall and drape vertically as if they were on a coat hanger. If you have ever tried to hang your clothes on a hanger that is too small or on a wire hanger that bends under the weight of a heavy garment, you know how clothes drape themselves on inadequate shoulders. It's great to have large shoulders; they don't need shoulder pads. But if you are self-conscious about them, there are tricks to downplay that area.

- Wear deep colors at the shoulder area. A good way to make your shoulders look less broad is to have your set-in sleeves darker than the rest of your top. A sleeveless tunic or vest over a deeper-colored bodice or T-shirt gives you the same result.

- Dropped sleeves will soften wide or angular shoulders, provided the fabric is soft and drapes nicely over your shoulders. The same style in a stiff or bulky fabric would have the contrary effect. Avoid gathered sleeves. Be careful with halter tops or cut-in armholes. They make your shoulders look wider.

- Set-in sleeves should not exceed your shoulder bones. You could even steal half an inch off your shoulder by setting your sleeves inside your shoulder bones. It is only a minor alteration for a good seamstress.

- Kimono, raglan, dolman, or dropped sleeves are better to soften square shoulders, providing the fabric is soft and drapable. As these sleeves don't have a seam at the shoulder edge, they don't require pads with a sharp edge. For these styles, you can use either softly rounded pads or no pads at all.

For more details, check the chart of the Gauguin shape in chapter 8.

HEAVY ARMS

- Avoid tight tops and sleeves. Sleeves that are too narrow create ugly horizontal lines in stiff fabrics, and rolls in knits.

- Loose sleeves are best for you. Have long sleeves tapered in toward the hemline.

- Beware of sleeves that are too short or sleeveless styles. Opt for long sleeves or sleeves that end just above or below the elbow. Raglan and dolman sleeves or dropped sleeves, if your shoulders are not sloping, give you enough ease and are cool in the warm season. Kimono and dolman sleeves are cut in one piece with the body and are always cut low under the arm, which will give enough room to an ample upper torso and to full arms. The raglan style also gives needed ease for your bust and arms. The diagonal shoulder seam of the raglan goes from neckline to underarm and has no shoulder edge seam (the deeper the diagonal cut, the fuller the sleeve). Beware, however, of extremely low-cut sleeves if you are short; they visually reduce your height.

- To divert attention from your challenges, create some center-front interest such as long strings of beads, oblong scarves, or center-front piping.

THIN ARMS

- Thin arms are only a problem if they are too thin in proportion to the rest of your body. They look better covered, at least down to the elbow. The biggest mistake is to wear short, full sleeves or short, cuffed sleeves. Those styles would make your arms look even thinner.

LARGE BREASTS

- Start with the right bra! A bra that gives your bosom an unflattering shape ruins the best outfit. See page 167.

- Keep your bust area as plain as possible. Forget about any eye-catching details in that area.

- Snug tops are absolute *no-nos*.

- Collars should be long, vertical, and narrow. Another option: choose collarless styles such as V neck or diagonals.

- If you have a shapely waist, wear belts, but blouse your tops, so as not to accentuate your ample bustline. Rubenesque shapes look better in dropped waistlines or unbroken vertical lines such as long tunics or loose dresses.

- Choose soft, drapable, but not too thin or clingy fabrics. Avoid stiff, bulky textures for your tops; they won't give you the desired streamlined look.

- Steer clear of large-scaled or widely spaced prints in a strong value contrast, such as black and white. Large- or medium-scaled prints should always have a subdued value contrast. Your best choices are solid-colored tops or dresses in a neutral or deep color.

- You can brighten up your tops and dresses with colorful scarves. Wear them hanging loose to create two vertical lines, which make your eye move up and down, or tie them low, below bust level.

- Wear your brooches high, near your shoulder area, to invite the eye close to your face, away from your bustline. Your necklaces should be either above or below your bust. A choker-length necklace, a necklace that ends just below the collarbone, or a long pendant that ends below the bustline are the best choices to make the eye pass over the challenge of your ample bust.

For more information, check your charts (Pop Art, Gauguin, Rubens) in chapter 8.

SMALL BREASTS

- Here again, it's only a challenge if your bottom half is heavy, as it is always a question of proportion and balance. Small busts can look very feminine. It's the shape of your bust that counts, not the size. Besides, it is easier to add a little extra than to downplay an impressive bustline.

- A good tip to balance an ample bottom is to add details at bust level. Breast pockets, large lapels, yokes, gatherings, horizontal seams, and layers all add the needed volume. Thick, crisp, or fuzzy textures help also. Gently bloused bodices will give the illusion of a fuller top.

For the appropriate bra, see "Underwear" on page 167.

WAISTS

Your waist separates the upper torso from the lower torso. On an average person, the distance from armpit to waist is equal to the distance from waist to crotch. The crotch should be at the midpoint between the top of your head and your feet.

Long Waist = Short Legs

- If you are long-waisted, your crotch will probably be lower than midway between the top of your head and your feet, and your legs will be shorter. The longer your waist, the shorter your legs. Hence, your challenge is short legs rather than a long torso. This is a problem that is easy to correct.

- ***Empire style is your very best choice!*** The high waist of this style gives the illusion of long legs, as you don't really see where your waist and bottom end. Skirts are better than pants for the same reason. If your waist can afford it, wear wide belts. Belts should always match the color below the waist as this adds some length to your legs. Match your hosiery and shoes with the color of your pants or skirts to visually lengthen the lower part of your body. Cuffed pants, hip huggers, or pants that are wide at the bottom are absolute no-nos.

- You might think that you should wear your skirt down to your ankles in order to lengthen your legs, but it will make your legs look shorter than they really are. The length of your skirt should not exceed one inch below your calf.

- Don't pair long jackets with long skirts. It will only weigh you down. Long skirts should be matched with short jackets. Remember, ***the shorter the top, the longer the bottom!*** For your jackets, choose high-waisted, semifitted styles. Bolero tops in a contrasting color will bring the eye up and horizontally divide a long torso.

- Always wear a narrow silhouette at your bottom half to lengthen that area. Stay away from too much texture and any details at hem level. It will visually shorten your lower torso.

- And, of course, wear shoes with heels to add some inches to your legs.

Short Waist = Long Legs

Are you short-waisted? That means you most probably have long legs, a great asset! Most pants and skirts and most skirt lengths will suit you. A short waist is only a challenge if your circumference is on the ample side, if you have a missing waist, or a low bustline. Even then, it is a challenge easy to correct by choosing the right length and proportion between your top and your bottom. All you have to do is visually lengthen your upper torso. The tips following tell you how to achieve this.

- Beware of belts! If you want to wear belts, select the narrow ones so as not to shorten the already limited space between waist and bustline. The color of your belts should match your tops. Contour belts are your best choice as the top of the belt sits below your waist. Overblouse your tucked-in tops to add some inches to your natural waistline. A hip sash is great if your hips allow it. But beltless styles suit you better and are less risky.

- Wear your jacket, vest, or tunic long. Select styles with dominant vertical lines for your tops. They should hang loose and straight for a streamlined, elongated look. Look for dropped waist styles to lengthen your upper torso. The same goes for dresses.

- Dresses are your best choice, as you don't really see where your upper torso ends. Opt for styles with unbroken vertical lines, such as a sheath, shift, princess dress, or coat dress. Monotone outfits optimize this unbroken vertical effect.

- Wear your tops long, but don't hide your assets, which are your long legs! Match your long top with a short skirt, rather than a long top with a long skirt. Remember, long in contrast to short lengthens, whereas short in contrast to long shortens. Keep the following formula in mind: *long tops + short bottoms for short waist and short tops + long bottoms for long waist.*

- Choose oblong scarves and wear them hanging loose to create vertical lines that will help to visually lengthen the upper torso.

STOMACH AND WAISTLINE

For an ample abdomen and waistline, follow the same principle already covered on this subject in chapter 8 in the chart for your body shape (Renoir, Rubens, Picasso). Here are just a few reminders.

- Don't tuck your tops into tight waistbands, and stay away from belts or any belted styles.

- Choose unstructured, long styles in soft, drapable fabrics for your tops, but beware of clingy, thin textures.

- Dresses such as sheaths, shifts, or single-breasted coat dresses with dominant, vertical lines are perfect to downplay the stomach area and to camouflage a missing waist.

- Avoid large-scaled, widely spaced prints or loud colors around abdomen area. Verticals or diagonals are best.

- Wear scarves and jewelry close to your face to bring the eye up, or look for oblong scarves and have them hang loose over your stomach. This, too, will create vertical lines.

- Beware of long pendants that swing and/or jiggle on your stomach every time you move. It will only focus attention to your challenging area.

AMPLE HIPS AND VOLUPTUOUS BUTTOCKS

Famous artists loved painting women with voluptuous buttocks and ample hips. I know it is a challenge to dress Rubenesque hips and buttocks, but here again, one can work around this challenge by strategically planning the right colors and values and by choosing the right fabrics to balance the proportions. Here are a few remainders to downplay that area.

- Always have your tops float over your butt and hips.

- Layer a tucked-in top with an open jacket.

- Make sure that the hemline of your tops does not end at the largest part of your bottom half, particularly if there is a strong color contrast between top and bottom items. This would create a horizontal line and, for sure, invite the eye across your butt.

- Select monochromatic outfits or choose a deeper shade for your skirts or pants.

- Never wear bulky or stiff fabrics over your curves. They make you look heavy and boxy, whereas soft, floating, curve-hugging fabrics will provide a streamlined silhouette.

- For narrow skirts and pants, look for styles with fabrics that contain a small percentage of stretch fibers for maximum comfort, such as Lycra or spandex. These fabrics give you maximum comfort, don't wrinkle, and are easy to care for (horizontal wrinkles in a tight skirt always make you look larger). Remember to match them with a long tunic or an open jacket.

- Skirts and pants without waistbands, which sit just below your waist, expose your curves less than a cinched waistband does.

- Forget about details below your waistline. Save them for your tops.

- Have the eye pass over your challenges by selecting lighter or stronger colors or vivid prints (with a scarf) close to your face.

HEAVY LEGS

- The right heel, the right skirt length, and the right hose can help to visually slenderize your legs.

- Always keep your skirts, hose, and shoes in a similar medium- to dark-toned value. Have them blend with each other. Strong contrasts would chop your legs horizontally and bring the eye down, where you don't want it. The same goes for details at the hemline.

- Make sure that your hemline is even to avoid bringing unwanted attention to your legs.

- Sheer or semiopaque hosiery helps to shadow your legs, which makes them look slimmer. In the warm season, wear nude-colored hose or none with light, bright, or pastel clothes. But steer clear of pastel-colored hosiery, even if they match your skirt. They would make your legs look even heavier.

- Heels will lengthen your legs. Choose a two- to three-inch heel, not too thin (spikes would not be in proportion to heavy legs), but a too-wide heel would look chunky.

- Look for shoes wide enough so they won't squeeze the flesh. Certain brands manufacture their shoes in different widths for each size. The letters A, B, and C correspond to the width. If your feet are wide, stay clear of shoes that have an A width. Don't ever believe that a shoe widens from wearing! If it does, it will lose its shape, too. The shoe has to fit your foot comfortably.

- T-strap styles divide your legs horizontally, and high openings shorten your foot by some inches. Small, dainty details or thin straps do not suit heavy legs. Your best buys are simple pumps without eye-catching details (you don't want to focus attention on your legs). Keep the décolleté (opening) of your shoes long and narrow, which visually lengthens your legs.

- Hem your skirts at the most flattering part of your legs. One inch up or down can make all the difference. Stand in front of a full-length mirror in your hose and shoes with the heel height you want to wear with your skirt. Hold your skirt in front of your legs (preferably a skirt that tones in with your hose). Start at your feet, and lift your skirt slowly until you find the length that suits your legs best, and most probably it will be one to two inches below the identation of your calf. The hemline should never end at the widest part of your calf.

THIN LEGS

Here again, thin legs as such are not a problem. It only becomes an issue if they are thin in proportion to a heavier body.

- Your worse mistake is to have too much texture at hem level. Your legs would only look lost, sticking out from a full skirt or wide or cuffed shorts.

- You will probably find your most flattering hem length is at the widest part of your calf or thigh, or just one to two inches above the knee. To find the right hem length for your legs, follow the same directions as in the "Heavy Legs" section.

- For you, opaque hosiery is better than sheer. Sheer hosiery shadows the outline of your legs and would make your legs look even thinner.

- Long skirts look best on you. Minis, shorts, and bermudas? Yes, as long as you keep the hemline narrow.

- Have fun with textured, patterned, and colored leggings! Wear them with socks or boots. It will give your skinny legs a more compact appearance. Don't wear heavy shoes without socks. Your thin legs would be out of proportion to your shoes.

- Low-cut shoes reveal thin legs less than high-cut ones.

PETITE AND VOLUPTUOUS

Being short is only an issue for robustly built women who are under five feet and over size 12.

A few years ago the clothes available for the petite but large woman were very limited. Nowadays you have good options in boutiques or in the petite section of department stores, where you can find trendy clothes with styles ranging from casual to classic.

The key element to look for is *an unbroken, elongating, streamlined silhouette*, with very few details, especially no eye-catching details below the waistline.

Stay clear of large-sized clothes that are not designed for petite women. Shortening alone is not a good enough solution. If you only shorten the outfit, it will always look unbalanced, the pockets will sit too low, buttons that start below bust level will end at the hemline, a back vent of a skirt or jacket will be too tiny or downright disappear, the crotch of pants will end down at your knees, collars will be too big in proportion to the outfit, and so on. You will spend a lot of money for needless alterations, and your outfit will still look out of proportion. Only simple styles with hardly any details can be considered for shortening, such as a simple sheath or shift with in-seam pockets, which can easily be raised. But in the end, you are better off with clothes that are designed for petite large women and thus are designed in proportion to your height.

Here are a few more tips to help you make the right choices.

SHAPES AND SILHOUETTE

Skirts and Pants

- Make sure that your skirts and pants have a narrow silhouette.

- Beware of ankle-length skirts if they are stiff, bulky, or wide at the bottom. Petite women tend to make the mistake of wearing maxi-length skirts, thinking this would elongate their figure, but it just makes them look like a small woman in clothes that are too big.

- Never cover your ankles, not even for an evening outfit.

- Mid-calf or just above or below the knee is a good skirt length for your height. A short skirt should always be tapered to avoid a boxy, square look.

- For a longer skirt, choose only soft, drapable fabrics, which will provide a narrow, flowing silhouette, as does knife or kick pleats in a knit or a soft, supple fabric.

- A-lined, gathered, tiered, or any full skirt with too much texture at the hemline will definitely make you look shorter.

- Narrow pants, such as stirrups, tapered, or straight-leg with a front pleat, help to elongate your figure.

- Stear clear of pant cuffs and hip huggers, which visually shorten your legs.

Tops and Dresses

- Take care not to wear shoulder pads that are too big as they give you a boxy appearance in proportion to your height.

- Tops that end below mid-thigh make your legs look shorter, unless you pair your top with a short skirt. A long jacket paired with a long skirt will overwhelm you and make you look even shorter. The maximum length of your top should not exceed twelve inches below your waist.

- Long tops are better teamed with pants or with skirts that are just above or just below knee level.

- Semifitted or loose styles (depending on your size) in fluid fabrics create a streamlined silhouette and elongate your figure.

- Beware of waist-fitted or body-contoured styles. These styles don't have a vertical drape, which gives an illusion of height.

- Wear your jackets unbuttoned to create a vertical center-front opening.

- For your dresses, choose narrow, fluid silhouettes. Loose-fitting styles, such as sheaths, shifts, dresses with a princess seam, or coat dresses, will suit you best. Stay clear of styles with dropped waistlines.

- Bloused tops and waist seams shorten your figure.

- If your upper arms are not too large, select styles with high armholes. Beware of dropped or dolman sleeves. Long, narrow sleeves are better than short ones. When shortening your sleeves, taper them to keep them narrow and in proportion to your height.

COLORS AND PRINTS

- Use colors and prints to bring the eye up. By adding interest to your top half, attention is drawn upward, which makes you appear taller. Eye-catching colors should be close to your face or even above. (Try a colorful beret with an eye-catching pin.)

- Monocolor outfits from head to toe will look best on you.

- Avoid contrasting colors between tops and bottoms, as this will break up your silhouette and create horizontal lines, which need to be avoided. If you really want color contrast, make sure to repeat the color from the bottom close to your face, or keep the top layer unbuttoned over a monochromatic outfit.

- Prints should be small to medium in scale and vertical in design. Avoid contrasting or widely spaced patterns, they only overload your figure.

- For separates, use small-scaled, all-over prints or prints on the top half only.

FABRICS

- Choose soft, drapable, smooth textures such as knits, jerseys, washed silk, crepes, challis, viscose and polyester blends, and rayon or a firmer texture such as gabardine, linen, or double jersey for a shift, sheath, or coat dress.

- Avoid fluffy, bulky, quilted, or stiff textures, as these fabrics will make you look boxy.

DETAILS

Skirts and Pants

- As you want to bring the eye up, stear clear of details below the waist, such as ruffles, flounces, open pleats, gathered yokes, patch pockets, and border prints or flounces at the hemline.

- Keep your skirts and pants as simple as possible, and save exciting details to focus attention to your top.

Tops and Dresses

- Opt for single-breasted tops with narrow front openings, lapels, and collars. If your bust is not too generous, a breast pocket with a hanky or colorful scarf helps to bring the eye up.

- Avoid strong horizontal lines, shoulder yokes, waist seams, or cuff details.

ACCESSORIES

Shoes

- Have your shoes match hose and skirt or pants.

- Choose pumps with a long décolleté, such as U- or V-shaped openings.

- A gently pointed toe will be more lengthening than a rounded or square one.

- Avoid T-straps, bows, or heavy buckles, so as not to create a horizontal effect.

- Beware of chunky, heavy boots and make sure the hem of your skirt covers the top of your boots to avoid empty space between boots and skirt, which will divide your legs horizontally and visually shorten your figure. Let your pants fall over your boots or tuck them into your boots, but only if pants and boots have the same color value.

- Do wear heels; it will add height. Reserve flat heels for narrow pants or minis only. Platform heels add length to your height, but make sure that they are not too heavy.

Handbags

- Your bags should be rather small. A big, bulky bag would be too overpowering for your petite figure.

- Keep your bags tone-in-tone with your shoes to avoid separate blocks of colors. Reserve bright colors to draw attention upward close to your face.

- Wear the strap of your bag short. You don't want the bag hanging down to your knees. Wear your bags above hip level, never below. It would make you look shorter.

Belts

- Avoid belts; they break the streamlined look of a garment, divide your silhouette horizontally, and make you look shorter.

Scarves

- Oblong scarves worn vertically create vertical lines and give you an elongated look.

- Avoid bulky scarves too close to your neck.

- Choose solid-colored scarves or scarves with a small- to medium-sized pattern. Here you can use eye-catching colors to bring the eye up.

Jewelry

- If you have to choose just one piece of jewelry, make it an earring or a hairpin to create a focal point as high as possible.

- Wear your brooches high.

- Have your necklaces end between collarbone and bust level (a short choker would disturb the desired open vertical neckline, and a long pendant would emphasize your petite scale in comparison).

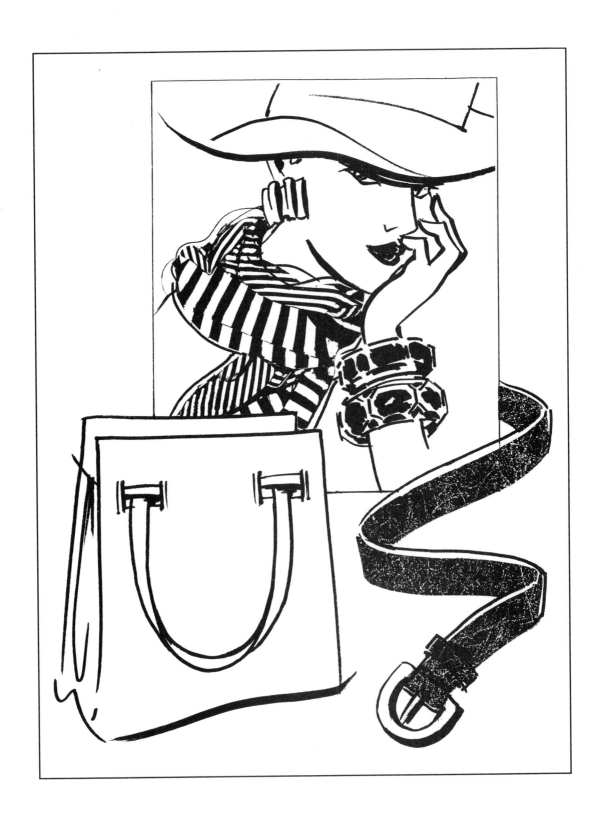

accessories

TEN GOOD REASONS TO WEAR ACCESSORIES

Accessories pull an outfit together and give it a final, very personal touch. They can be your signature. Combining accessories with your clothes opens up endless possibilities to express moods and create different looks and styles. Depending upon the way you coordinate them with your clothes, you can achieve different effects. Accessories can create balance, add sizzle to a garment, can pull an outfit together, transform it, update it, contrast or complement it, and a lot more.

1. **Accessories can lead the viewer's eye to your assets.** A choker necklace or drop-style earrings will draw attention to a long neck. A contrasting colored belt will highlight a tiny waist, a hip sash will enhance slender hips, and textured hose will show off long, shaply legs.
2. **Accessories can relate different items of your outfit to each other.** If you wear a black skirt with a white top, you can relate them to each other by a patterned scarf that contains both colors.
3. **Accessories can add an exciting element to an otherwise sober facade.** Some bold earrings or necklaces, a scarf in a strong accent color, a colorful hanky for your breast pocket, or a lovely knotted tie or scarf in an intense color can transform an ordinary outfit into an extraordinary one. But don't overdo it. Less is more!
4. **Accessories can dress an outfit up or down.** A simple black dress can be transformed into an evening dress by wearing a precious shawl, a scarf made out of velvet, *iridescent hose* (FOR WELL-SHAPED LEGS ONLY), pumps in a metallic shade, a jeweled buckle on a belt, or dressy

jewelry. Conversely, the same dress paired with a sporty shoulder bag, a handwoven textured scarf, a leather belt with rustic topstiching, or sporty loafers will change it into a casual dress.

5. **Accessories can underline your personal style.** If you are the classic type and would like to accentuate that style, you will most probably opt for more conservative accessories, such as a string of pearls, precious gold or silver jewelry, diamond studs, a Hermés scarf, a Chanel or Gucci type of handbag (they can be knockoffs, as long as they don't pretend to be real). Whereas an earthy, outdoor person will look best in ethnic jewelry in natural materials, such as wood, leather, or stone, handwoven scarves, shoulder or tote bags in canvas, straw, or leather.

6. **Accessories can change the mood of an outfit.** A strict, masculine suit can be given femininity by wearing a lacy scarf or a breast-pocket hanky, a few layers of pearls, or both, whereas feathers and boas can add a flirtatious touch and high heels can turn your suit into a seductive outfit.

7. **Accessories can make a garment look expensive.** An expensive leather belt or a sophisticated shawl or scarf can upgrade an inexpensive garment, whereas a cheap plastic belt, run-down heels, or a cheap nylon or acrylic scarf will ruin any outfit.

8. **Accessories can update an outfit.** Play around with trendy fantasy jewelry to update a garment. Such jewelry is inexpensive, so you can throw it away the following season. A scarf in a trendy color or pattern will also update any basics.

9. **Accessories help to create balance.** Repeating the color of your hose or shoes with a scarf will lead the eye up and down, visually elongate your figure, and create a color balance between top and bottom.

10. **Accessories can counter your challenge.** A shawl, a beret in a strong color, or jewelry close to your face will invite the eye up, away from voluptuous curves at the bottom area. Conversely, patterned or colored hose (for shapely legs only) will help to divert attention from an ample upper torso.

SHOES

When buying a pair of shoes, your first criterion should be comfort, and comfort means quality. Only buy good-quality shoes. Yes, they are expensive, but it is not a luxury (buy your classics on sale). Quality shoes are made out of soft leather and don't just exist in different sizes; you can also find them in various widths. The letters A to C relate to the breadth of your foot. A shoe in a high-quality leather and the right width adapts to the form of your foot, whereas a foot will never adapt to your shoe. Cheap shoes will also wear out fast, whereas expensive shoes can be resoled a few times before you will need to buy a new pair.

Choosing appropriate footwear is extremely important as it does influence the general look of your outfit and the way you walk. The wrong shoe or, more precisely, the wrong height of a heel, can ruin a silhouette. The wrong style or color will conflict with your clothes and destroy any look. For instance, a comfy pair of heavy-soled shoes defuse the look of a business outfit. The best outfit can be spoiled by a scuffed shoe, a run-down heel, or a cheap, plastic soled shoe.

TIP: New shoes with leather soles last much longer if you take them to a shoemaker to have a thin rubber sole added to protect the leather sole.

Style

For a casual style, you just can't go wrong with classics such as mocassins, loafers, or Oxfords. They come in flat to medium-high heels and are appropriate at work, too. A pair of pumps should definitely be part of your footwear. They are always in fashion, adapt to any style, and can be worn at any occasion. Look for narrow, low-cut V or U openings to slenderize your legs and foot. Wear closed pumps for a tailored suit or a more professional look. Open-toe styles, such as sandals or a slingback, better balance light, fluid, transparent, or gauzy clothes. The less detail on a shoe, the better. Avoid shoes with unusual toe shapes, such as too pointed, too square, or very round shapes. They are fashionable today and outdated tomorrow.

If your legs need slimming, avoid heavy, chunky shoes, as well as ones that are too delicate. The first will make your legs look even heavier, and the second would just emphasize the breadth of your legs. Ankle straps only look good with delicate ankles.

Women with long feet should avoid excessively pointed shoes. With pointed shoes you always have to choose a larger size to give room for your toes. This would add unwanted length to an already long foot. Low-cut shoes visually lengthen a leg but shorten a long foot. Conversely, high-cut shoes shorten a leg but lengthen a foot. An extended sole also adds inches to your foot.

Boots

Except for snow boots, boots don't need to be heavy. There is a large choice of great boots available today. Ankle boots with a flat to medium-high heel are a perfect choice with pants. For skirts that end just below mid-calf, a boot should be slightly higher so the hemline of your skirt will cover the top of your boot. Never have a gap between your boots and your skirt, as this would divide your legs horizontally, visually shorten them, and break up height. Of course, this does not apply to boots paired with a miniskirt if your legs are well-shaped and worth showing. High boots look best with a flat to medium-high heel.

Heels

Heels are tricky. They can make or break a silhouette. The wrong heel with the wrong clothes will ruin the overall proportion of your silhouette and throw you out of balance. An outdated heel can spoil a trendy outfit.

When selecting the height and the width of a heel, you should consider the shape and size of your legs, the hem length of your outfit, and the width of your outfit at hem level.

If your legs are on the heavy side, avoid stocky heels, such as a wedge or a platform; they make your legs look broader. So do thin, stiletto heels, as they make a stark contrast with robustly shaped legs. Stilettos also unattractively accentuate skinny legs.

Wear your heels just high enough to allow you to keep a gracious gait.

Advice for selecting the right height of a heel:

- Texture at hem level, as is the case with palazzo pants, bell-bottoms, wide, straight pants, or gathered, ankle-length skirts, need a heel to offset and lift the weight of all that texture. Avoid flat heels with heavy, ankle-length textures as they weigh you down (unless you are very tall).

- Flats look fine with narrow pants or a mini, and, if you are tall, a long, narrow skirt.

- Select flats with a flexible sole, such as natural latex. They give you a more gracious stride than a shoe with a hard, synthetic sole.

Colors

Keep expensive shoes in neutral colors so they match with most items of your wardrobe. This way you can wear them for years. Trendy, unusual colors, such as lime green or orange, outdate very fast. They are not worth the price per wearing. But if you find some trendsetters at a good price, and they are comfortable, go ahead and have fun!

Never wear white shoes, except sneakers and jogging shoes! White shoes make a foot look bigger. In summer, choose oat, beige, or light taupe shades instead; they match white, pastel, and neutral clothes.

Bright colors in shoes are sheer luxury. They are difficult to match with most of your wardrobe. However, they can bring pizzazz to your dresses and bring attention to shapely legs and small feet.

Please don't select your shoes and handbag in the same accent color. It is outlandish and just contrived. You can, but don't have to, coordinate shoes with your handbag as long as the colors are neutral (except white). Do, however, keep your shoes in the same or slightly darker tone than your hose. **"Your legs look longer when the color of your shoes doesn't act like a stop sign."** (Marlene Dietrich, who always wore matching hosiery, quoted by Patty Fox in her book *Star Style*).

HOSIERY

Shoes should never be lighter than your hose, except for a bare-colored hose. Dark, sheer pantyhose shadows the outline of your legs and makes them look thinner. Keep a second pair in your handbag; a run in your hose is an instant image breaker. Avoid a dark, sheer hose if you have pronounced calf muscles but thin ankles. Sheer stockings will shadow your ankles more than your calves and thereby emphasize your calves in contrast.

Lace or patterned hose do not flatter any type of legs, and net stockings can look vulgar. Never wear white or pastel hosiery. They make your legs look heavy and unsexy. Wear a bare shade hose for light clothes only.

Keep opaque hosiery for sporty shoes, sheer hose for dressy occasions. Textured hose looks great on shapely or skinny legs with a short skirt. For cold weather, you can add some woolen socks with your sporty shoes or some leg warmers rolled over your boots.

HANDBAGS

A handbag is expensive, and you don't want to change it every season. A top-quality bag in a classic style and a neutral color is a wise choice and a long-term investment, and it can be used throughout the year.

When selecting a bag, you should also take into consideration your size and personal style. For instance, an outdoor person needs a more casual bag, such as a shoulder bag, knapsack, or a tote in soft leather. A more structured, classic tote works better for a career woman.

Always choose your handbag in proportion to your shape. A large bag on a petite woman looks as out of proportion as a delicate bag on an impressive figure. If you are short in height, shorten your shoulder bag strap so your bag doesn't hang down to your knees and make you look even shorter. Ideally, a bag should not hang lower than your hips.

Coordinate your bag with your clothes. A handbag with an accent color can add a flicker of flamboyance to an outfit but visually disrupt the height of a silhouette. So avoid it if your are short.

If your body is on the generous side, avoid bulky styles, such as a bulky knapsack or an overly loaded tote. It only adds additional width.

A bag does not have to match the color of your shoes or your outfit, but it should be coordinated with the look and mood of your clothes, or, even better, accentuate it for an overall put-together look, just like any other accessory. Don't match a sophisticated, precious pearl necklace with a sporty bag or pair a structured, professional looking bag with a polka-dot dress; it would diffuse the nostalgic look of the dress.

An everyday bag has to be practical and versatile. The shape should be timeless, medium-scaled (rather flat), in a good, soft, quality leather and in a neutral shade that will blend in with most of your clothes. A medium-sized tote, a shoulder bag, or a knapsack are the best choices for an everyday bag. A tote can look professional, sporty, or even elegant, depending on the material and finishing used. A shoulder bag comes in a sporty or a more feminine, Chanel-type version. It can even be used for the evening, as a modern and younger alternative to an envelope clutch. A knapsack is a sporty, stylish version of a shoulder bag. You can wear it on your back or over your shoulder. A belt bag is great for traveling or shopping when you need both hands to carry your luggage or groceries. Wear it loosely around your waist.

What about a bag with a handle? Unless you are very young, with a sure, subtle flare for the latest trend, or have the courage to wear it with a funky outfit, pass on this style. To me, a bag with a handle will always have that outlandish look, as it is not really in tune with the times, or, more precisely, in tune with a modern woman's lifestyle. But, if you love the look, have it as an extra bag. To counter that tight, fussy look, wear a modern, casual hairstyle with it.

Whatever style you use for your bag, go for quality. Avoid shiny materials, eye-catching buckles, and complicated, overly decorative details. It gives a bag a cheap and outdated look and makes it more difficult to match with your clothes. For the summer, you can look for a more inexpensive bag in canvas, straw, or sailcloth.

Once you have your everyday bag in a neutral color and you fall in love with a brightly colored bag, go ahead, buy it! It will brighten up any neutral outfit and looks especially dramatic with black. Just, please, don't ever think of matching it with the same-colored shoes! Two focus points below your waist will unbalance your silhouette. Besides, as I already mentioned, coordinating shoes and handbag in the same strong color is outdated.

BELTS, SCARVES, SHAWLS, AND HATS

Belts

Belts can change the shape and proportion of a silhouette. Strategically used, they can visually lengthen a short waist or, conversely, shorten a long waist. Belts, just as any other accessories, can give an outfit a finished look, transform it, update it, create balance, or change the whole mood or look of it.

- If you are tall and slim, you can wear any belt. It can be large or narrow, in a neutral or bold color. You can buckle it tightly or loosely at the waist, or have it fall below the waistline. You can wear a waist sash to show off a slim waist or a hip sash to focus attention to slender hips. The choices are endless.

- Belts interrupt the vertical drape of an outfit, divide a silhouette horizontaly, and are therefore not recommended for heavy women, unless you follow certain guidelines:

    1. Wear your belts under an open jacket only.
    2. The color of your belt should blend into the color of your clothes.
    3. Keep your belt narrow.
    4. Never clinch your belt too tightly, as this will make your stomach bulge out.
    5. Buckle a belt loosely enough that it falls lower in the front, which will create a slight V line at your tummy.
    6. Overblouse your tops gently.

- If you are long-waisted, the belt should match the color of your clothes below the waist to add length to your lower torso. If you are short-waisted, match the color of your belt with your top to visually lengthen the upper torso (for more details see the section on waists on page 181.)

- If your skirt, pants, or dress comes with a plastic belt, replace it with a good-quality leather belt or get rid of the belt and belt loops. Clothes with belt loops always look unfinished without a belt.

- Dark-colored belts are better than light ones, as they visually slenderize your waist.

- Wear contrasting-colored belts only if your waist is an asset.

- Buy expensive belts in neutral colors, as with bags and shoes, such as black, brown, burgundy, navy, taupe, and tan. Only one with a tiny waist can allow herself the luxury of a belt in an accent color to spice up a classic outfit and create a focal point in that area.

- Avoid an overly decorated buckle or belt for daytime wear. It risks looking cheap and often clashes with the look of your clothes. Conversely, for a dressy occasion, you can scatter some studs or pins on a plain belt or replace a simple buckle with a jeweled one to turn it into a precious piece. You could also create your own belt by turning a large pendant or a brooch into a buckle. Have the old buckle removed and replace it with a press button (a shoemaker can do that easily). Cover the press button with a large jewel or a precious badge. It will be your own creation. Again, this is only recommended for women who want to focus attention to their waistline.

Scarves and Shawls

A scarf is one of the most popular, practical, and versatile accessories. You can use it as a head wrap, a neckline accent, a necklace, a tie, or an ascot. You can make a belt out of it, such as a waist wrap or a hip sash. In no time, you can turn a scarf into a halter top, a sun wrap, or a sarong. You can even change it into a pouch. You can use it for work, weekends, and evenings. There are endless possibilities to create different looks, depending on the size, shape, fabric, and print of a scarf.

Colors

A colorful scarf is the easiest and most inexpensive way

- to spice up an outfit

- to bring out a color in a print of your clothes

- to relate different colors of your separates

- to create a focus point, hence divert attention from your figure problems

- to use it as a balance strategy (see page 191).

As long as they suit your skin tone, have fun with brightly colored scarves, such as yellow, orange, red, and shocking pink, or try intensive jewel tones such as emerald, topaz, turquoise, cardinal red, jade, gold, amber, and chrome. They look really striking when worn with deeper shades.

Scarves in pale shades add a delicate, feminine touch and look expecially sophisticated when paired with light neutrals. Try cool pastels such as silver, light aqua, mint, lavender, and orchid if you have a cool skin tone and warm pastels such as cream, peach, apricot, salmon, melon, or shell pink for a warm skin tone.

Patterns

Scarves come in many different patterns or jacquards (woven-in patterns). You have the choice between geometrics, checks and stripes, abstract prints, floral prints, exotic prints, or ethnic prints. A patterned scarf can always be matched with a solid-colored outfit, and if you have an innate flair, pair it with one or more prints that have the same color combination.

Texture

For extra flair, try visual contrast in texture only, such as a combination of shiny and matte, or rough and smooth. For instance, coordinate a soft, flowing, shiny satin scarf tone-in-tone with a matte wool crepe dress, or a nubby, open-weave cotton scarf with a smooth, shimmery silk top.

When shopping for a scarf, look for soft, drapable, and fluid textures for easy handling. The back side of your scarves should look equally pretty so that you can knot, loop, and tie them the way you want.

- Hold one corner of a square scarf and check how it falls on the bias.

- Tie it in a knot to make sure it does not bulk.

- Hold it against your skin and see how it feels.

Here are some recommended fabrics: chiffon, wool challis, cashmere, knits, twill, charmeuse, and velvet.

Choose scarves that are flakey, airy, fuzzy, furry, smooth, silky, wooly, satiny, lacy, warm, and soft. Avoid scarves that have stiff, crisp, rough, rigid, thick, coarse, or dense textures.

A Few More Tips

- Learn to wear scarves in a casual way.

- A scarf has to flatter your complexion.

- A scarf should project your personality.

- Always fold square scarves diagonally.

- Anchor a shawl with a brooch, a pin, or a hidden safety pin to avoid constant readjustment.

- A scarf should not draw attention to itself but should enhance your face and outfit.

- Check out store window displays or study fashion magazines to learn how stylists twist, knot, or tie a scarf.

- Do look into the men's section of a department store for scarves in classic prints and extra length.

- The busier the scarf, the simpler the outfit should be.

- Beware of large shawls if you are small; they can be overpowering.

- Matching a color below the waistline to the color of a scarf close to your face creates a color balance.

- If your neck is short or heavy, an oblong scarf is preferable to a square one. Tie or knot it low or let it hang loose.

- If you are a hat person, turn a scarf into a head wrap.

To learn all the different ways to twist, tie, loop, and knot a scarf, consult the fabulous little book *Sensational Scarves* by Carol Straley. It will give you simple, step-by-step instructions to make scarf dressing really fun.

Hats

Do you enjoy being noticed? Do you have a stylish flair and a casual attitude? Then go ahead and express yourself with a hat and have fun. But if you feel self-conscious in hats, you are better off without one. *How* you wear a hat is more important than the hat itself. A hat worn the wrong way or paired with conservative clothes can look very outlandish and give you a stiff, ladylike look. But a hat worn nonchalantly can add pizzazz and give you that special something, that casual sophistication. Like any other accessory, a hat has to match the look of your clothes. It can add to a mysterious, theatrical, or dramatic look, can look sophisticated, sporty, classic, funky, or romantic (romantic does not mean ultradelicate or dainty). Whatever the look, a hat should, and certainly does, make a strong statement and therefore asks for a strong personal style.

If you are daring enough to wear an outstanding hat, keep the style of your clothes simple. Don't go full tilt everywhere.

Style

A beret is the most practical and versatile, the most timeless, and the easiest to wear of all hats. It suits most lifestyles, occasions, and looks. It's soft and light but gives you warmth. It looks casual, natural, and young. It comes in all different looks and textures. Choose tweeds and corduroy for a sporty outdoor look, wool flannel for an everyday look. A beret made out of brocade, taffeta, or velvet is dressy and looks great with evening wear.

A beret is the perfect choice for small women, as it creates a focal point above your face and therefore adds height to a silhouette without overpowering a delicate figure.

And now some other classics, which will need more courage to wear. Try a cowboy hat, a Southwestern hat, or a Panama for a casual, sporty look. A fedora, a derby, a breton, or a boater are better paired with elegant sporty clothes. If you are tall, have fun with a portrait (very large, soft brim) for a dramatic look. A hat with a veil or a boa gives a flirtatious look.

Brims should never be larger than your shoulders. Here again, it's a matter of proportion. A hat with a brim that is too wide will make you look shorter instead of adding height to your figure.

Keeping your hat tone-in-tone with your clothes adds length to your silhouette. But hats in an accent color, if not too big, add panache to a neutral outfit, bring the eye up, and therefore lengthen, too. Wearing the same color for shoes and hat creates a color balance, inviting the eye to dance up and down a visually elongated silhouette. But please keep it quiet between head and toe.

JEWELRY

It is the jewelry that reveals the type of woman you are and the style you prefer. You could be any of the following style types, or even a combination:

- Discreet-Elegant

- Chic-Conservative

- Dramatic-Flamboyant

- Bohemian-Artistic

- Romantic-Delicate

Jewelry, just like perfume, is something very personal, very unique. That's why most women prefer to select their own jewelry.

Choose your jewelry carefully, give it a place of honor, and wear it appropriately. Jewelry will then enhance your assets and brighten up your face but not focus attention to itself alone. Jewelry, just like any other accessory, should relate to your style type and build, as well as to the occasion for which it is worn. Whatever your style, you should own at least one or two pieces of jewelry in a simple, distinct design. It will go with everything, you can wear it anywhere, and it lasts forever. But beware! Don't waste your money on precious metals or gems in a tacky design. You are better off with a less-expensive but well-designed piece.

Wear jewelry that is right for your body only. For instance:

- Shoulder lusters (excessively long, dangling earrings that literally touch the shoulder) only look good on a long, slender neck.

- Wear chokers (necklaces that are worn fitted around the neck) only if your neck allows it.

- Stay clear of long pendants (ornaments placed on a long chain or string) if your stomach protrudes.

- Avoid brooches if your bust is too generous.

- Bold, oversized jewelry close to your face demands a strong face, whereas a delicate piece asks for fine features.

- Don't pile rings on your fingers if your fingers are short and/or well fleshed.

Jewelry, like any other accessory, has to be in scale with your build. Tiny pieces on a Rubenesque figure would be lost and would only emphasize an impressive build. Conversely, big, bold pieces overpower a delicate figure.

Jewelry has to be appropriate for different occasions. Glittery, bold, or noisy pieces are not appropriate in a corporate environment. They don't make you look very professional. One or two strands of pearls or beads, gold or silver jewelry in a simple design, or precious or semi-precious stones in a distinctive setting are always a safe choice for work.

Additional Tips

- Jewelry doesn't really need to match exactly in design, but if you wear more than one piece at a time, make sure they match with each other in style and mood.

- Matching a specific design as a set (pin, necklace, earrings, and bracelets) gives you a tight and fussy look.

- Two or more outstanding pieces worn at a time only compete with each other. One eye-catching piece is enough.

- You can mix different metals, such as gold and silver, but only when they are combined in one piece of jewelry. However, don't mix a gold brooch with a silver choker. They just don't relate to each other.

- Make sure your jewelry does not interfere with ornamental buttons on a blouse or a jacket.

- Don't bother wearing a precious, delicate piece of jewelry on a loud, aggressive print; it won't be noticed.

- Trendy pieces can update an outfit in no time, but don't spend too much on them since they outdate fast.

- Looking like a chandelier risks appearing rather flashy!

- An elegant look is always spare and sober.

- Poorly designed jewelry always looks cheap.

- Wearing jewelry as a badge of wealth merely makes you look vulgar.

- Jangling, noisy pieces of jewelry are disturbing to you and those around you.

- A striking piece of jewelry can turn the simplest outfit into a sensational one.

- A modern piece of jewelry can add sizzle to an otherwise sober facade.

- When wearing a stunning, oversized piece, keep the outfit simple to tone down the drama of the jewelry.

- For a work-into-dressy change, wear nothing but a necklace or pendant on bare skin under your suit. It will add a sensual touch and, more important, make the necessary transformation in your appearance.

- Warm-toned metals, such as gold or copper, flatter women with a warm skin tone, and cool metals, such as white gold or silver, brighten up a cool-toned complexion.

A Look That's Uniquely Yours

Be daring! Use your jewelry out of context; use it in an unexpected way—**your way**! The result could be a great surprise! For instance:

- An earring or a brooch can be turned into an ornamental pendant.

- Take a clip-on earring and clip it into a buttonhole or onto a breast pocket.

- A few studs scattered on a belt can turn your waist into a focus point.

- A dressy hairpin can be used as a brooch.

- A decorative ear clip can be clipped on a lapel.

- A hair clip can keep your wrap skirt or shawl in place.

- If your thighs are well shaped, you can scatter some studs on your leggings or jeans.

- You can pin, clip, or sew a brooch or studs on a velvet ribbon to turn it into a unique choker.

- You can change a precious button into a cluster earring by glueing a clip on the back.

Indeed, creativity has no limits, and I'm sure you can explore many more possibilities to create your own conversation piece.

epilogue

You have now discovered the fundamentals of, and acquired a natural instinct for, dressing slim. You know how to dress in harmony with your own body shape and how to slenderize your silhouette. Having an in-depth understanding of timeless dressing fundamentals (which are to fashion what scales are to music), you will increase tenfold your ability to dress in style. When you are in doubt, consult this book.

What about fashion trends? To answer this question, let's return for a moment to the concept of style. In fashion, style is influenced by collective and personal factors.

Collective factors include culture, social styles, and trends. What is considered commonplace in New York, London, or Paris may be considered provocative somewhere else. Social styles lead some women to prefer classics, whereas others choose sophistication, nostalgia, avant-garde, romanticism, or a sporty look. Trends materialize in seasonal collections of fashion designers. You don't have to consider them as a must, but trust the words of fashion designer Karl Lagerfeld, who said in 1997 on American television, "We don't try to impose anything, we make proposals, only proposals. Of course we hope that they will please and we are very proud when they do, but ultimately the women will tell which design they prefer and which trend they favor."

At the other end of the spectrum, there is you, your personal choice, **your uniqueness**.

Balance all these factors, be modern, and above all, be yourself.

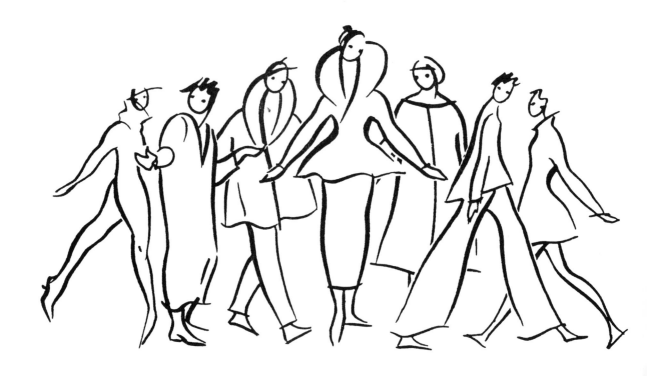

INDEX